Susan Lasher

Stop Treating Symptoms and Start Resolving Trauma!

Inside-Out Healing for Survivors of ALL Types

by

Denice Adcock Colson
M.S., L.P.C., C.T.R.T.

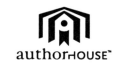

authorHOUSE™

1663 LIBERTY DRIVE, SUITE 200
BLOOMINGTON, INDIANA 47403
(800) 839-8640
WWW.AUTHORHOUSE.COM

This book is a work of non-fiction. Names of people and places have been changed to protect their privacy.

© *2004 Denice Adcock Colson M.S., L.P.C., C.T.R.T.*
All Rights Reserved.

No part of this book may be reproduced, stored in a retrieval system, or transmitted by any means without the written permission of the author.

First published by AuthorHouse 09/27/04

ISBN: 1-4184-8483-0 (e)
ISBN: 1-4184-8481-4 (sc)
ISBN: 1-4184-8482-2 (dj)

Library of Congress Control Number: 2004096387

Printed in the United States of America
Bloomington, Indiana

This book is printed on acid-free paper.

Acknowledgment

"I'll tell you what it really means to worship the LORD, Remove the chains of prisoners who are chained unjustly. Free those who are abused! Share your food with everyone who is hungry; share your home with the poor and homeless. Give clothes to those in need; don't turn away your relatives. Then your light will shine like the dawning sun, and you will quickly be healed. Your honesty will protect you as you advance, and the glory of the LORD will defend you from behind. When you beg the LORD for help, he will answer, 'Here I am!'" Isaiah 58:6-9. CEV

I want to thank Jesse Collins and Nancy Carson for all of their hard work and self-less dedication to developing this wonderful model and answering all of my tedious questions.

I also want to thank Craig Carson who first introduced me to ETM through his workshop in Houston, Texas, and trained me to be a trainer.

"It takes a lot of courage to show your dreams to someone else." – Erma Bombeck

Thanks Guys!!

Warning—Disclaimer

This book is intended to furnish information in reference to the subject matter recorded. It is sold with the assumption that the author and publisher are *not*, through this book, *providing therapy, counseling, legal or other professional services*. If therapy or other expert assistance is required, *please seek the services of a competent professional.*

It is not the aim of this work to reprint all the data that is otherwise available to the author and/or the publisher but to add to the already vast amount of information already in print. You are encouraged to read all of the accessible material. Learn as much as possible about the effects of trauma and resolving those effects. Tailor the information to your individual needs.

Every attempt has been made to construct this work in as complete and accurate a fashion as possible. However, there may be typographical and content errors. Therefore, this book should be utilized only as a guide and not as the absolute source of resolving past trauma. In addition, this work contains information on trauma resolution only up to the printing date.

The aim of this text is to inform and entertain. The author and Trauma Education & Consultation Publishing shall have neither liability nor responsibility to any entity or person with reference to any loss or damage caused, or purported to be caused, directly or indirectly by the data contained in this book.

If you do not wish to be constrained by the previous agreement, you may return this text to the publisher for a complete refund.

Table of Contents

Acknowledgment v
Warning—Disclaimer vii
Introduction xiii

CHAPTER ONE: INTRODUCING ETIOTROPIC TRAUMA MANAGEMENT AND TRAUMA RESOLUTION THERAPY 1

    What Makes ETM Different? 2
    Differences between TRT and Other Helping Relationships 4
    Specific Differences between TRT/ETM and Other Helping Models? 5
    Integrating Christian Faith with Trauma Resolution Therapy ... 9

CHAPTER TWO: UNDERSTANDING THE INFLUENCE TRAUMA HAS HAD ON YOUR LIFE 11

    Patterns of Trauma 12
        Initial Effects 12
        Life-Long Effects 13
        Initial Effects 14
        Life-Long Effects 14
        Initial Effects 15
        Life-Long Effects 15
    The Pre-Trauma Personal Identity of the Individual 16
    The Post-Trauma Personal Identity of the Individual 19
        Post-Trauma Existential Component of Personal Identity 19
    Post-Trauma Operational Component of Personal Identity 25

CHAPTER THREE: THE EFFECT OF TRAUMA ON FAMILIES AND OTHER RELATIONSHIPS 31

    First Incident 33
    Second Incident 36
    Third Incident 39
    The Chemically Dependent Perpetrator and Projection 42
    The Trauma Victim and Projection 43

CHAPTER FOUR: SURVIVAL RESPONSES—A DIFFERENT WAY OF LOOKING AT SYMPTOMS 47

    The Impact on Self-image.. 54
    Multiple Sources of Trauma 55
    Survival Responses or Sin?.. 58
    Religious Myths about Emotional Healing 60

CHAPTER FIVE: COMPLETING TRAUMA RESOLUTION THERAPY—THE FIVE PHASE PROCESS AND HOW IT IS DONE.. 63

    Phase One: The Written Component.. 65
        Exceptions... 68
        Examples of Other Phase One Incidents..................................... 69
    The Reading Process 72
    Phase Two... 77
    Phase Three 81
    Phase Four.. 83
    Phase Five A 85
    Phase Five B 87

CHAPTER SIX: WHAT DOES TRT ACCOMPLISH?...................... 89

    What to Expect 92
        Initial Effects.. 92
        Life-Long Effects.. 92

CHAPTER SEVEN: FORGIVENESS AND TRT 99

    Forgiveness Myths... 103
    Forgiveness and the Cycle of Grief.. 105

CHAPTER EIGHT: MARRIAGE AND FAMILY COUNSELING DURING THE TRAUMA RECOVERY PROCESS 109

    TRT Couples' Counseling With Addicts...111
    Counseling with Couples When the Trauma is in the Past........112
    More Advanced Marriage Counseling 112

CHAPTER NINE: USING TRT WITH ADOLESCENTS AND CHILDREN 117

    Children..117
    Adolescents..118
    Adolescents in Traumatized Families 120

    Working with the Parents of Abusive Adolescents and Young Adults 121

CHAPTER TEN: ADDICTION AS A PERPETRATOR 123

CHAPTER ELEVEN: ETM FOR CRISIS MANAGEMENT PERSONNEL AND ORGANIZATIONS 133

    Military Personnel 141

CHAPTER TWELVE: VICTORY! TRUE STORIES OF PEOPLE OVERCOMING TRAGEDY IN THEIR LIVES 143

    Anna 143
    Sarah 144
    Dana 145
    Bob and Alice 146
    Janice 146
    Nora 147
    Bethany 148
    Terry and David 148
    Mark 149
    Barbara 149
    Karen 150

APPENDIX A: TRAUMA ASSESSMENT 153

    As a child: 153
    As an adult (answer the previous questions as well as the following): 154

APPENDIX B: ETIOTROPIC TRAUMA MANAGEMENT FAQ'S 157

ENDNOTES 163

Introduction

Have you ever felt stuck? Either in your own personal counseling or in working with a client, just stuck? In 1992, I was working with a client in my office and she had the boldness to say to me "Denice, you have helped me a lot, but I just feel stuck." I was honest in return and said "I agree. You are stuck. And, honestly, I don't know what to do about it." Since she was a Christian I continued "But, let's pray about it and ask God to show us what to do next. I'm sure He will." We prayed right then and each went our separate ways. Sadly, I didn't give it another thought.

Within the week, the marketing director at the hospital where my psychiatrist partner and I had a Christian inpatient program approached me and asked him and me to attend a "Trauma Resolution Therapy" workshop being hosted by the hospital the following week. Marketing Directors can be very persuasive and, against my will, I found myself sitting in that workshop a week later. My attitude was one of "Just try to teach me something!" In spite of my attitude, he did! It wasn't until the third day, however, that the Holy Spirit was able to break through my pride and show me that THIS was the answer to the simple prayer my client and I had prayed only a week or so earlier. By the end of the week I knew I would not only be using TRT in my own practice, but that someday I would be teaching others how to use it in their ministries.

After the seminar I immediately started two TRT groups in my outpatient office and began using the TRT education program in our inpatient center. Within a few months I had a third group going and I have never looked back. Not once has TRT, when followed correctly, failed to resolve the trauma in a person who has completed all five phases.

After a number of years of training others, I finally had the opportunity to go through my own five-phase process on my own trauma. Although I had watched others experience the emotions, the pain, and then the release, when I went through it myself, I was even more sold on this process. Until I had completed the process, I was not fully aware of how much my past trauma had consumed my mind and affected my life. After completing phase 5, it was as if it evaporated into space. Sure, I can recall it if I try, but I have to put effort into bringing it to memory. Reliving the emotions connected to the memory became not only extremely difficult, but not worth the effort. I can honestly say that the self-esteem, confidence, sensitivity, sense of purpose and feeling of connection to God that had been stolen from me were fully restored. It's as if I came back to myself; back to the person I was prior to the trauma occurring. I wasn't even aware of how far I had strayed from my *self* until I completed the process.

Contrary to much popular opinion, the way in which you are affected by trauma has nothing to do with your education, your intelligence, your spiritual maturity or your character. It has to do with your brain. Trauma affects your brain. Traumatic incidents cause neurobiological changes in your brain over which you have no control. Alas, we all have frail human brains that are affected by trauma the same way. It's not your fault. You can't prevent it from happening to you nor can you make the damage go away through force of will. You don't have to have been diagnosed with Post Traumatic Stress Disorder in order to have been affected, either. If trauma has happened in your life, it affected your brain.

Trauma can be resolved naturally (without professional counseling), as you will read later in this book. But unfortunately, external things get in the way of that resolution for many people. As you begin to learn what it means to "think Etiotropically", you will see that we treat trauma because it happened, not because of the symptoms.

My prayer for you as you read this book—whether you are a survivor of trauma feeling stuck in your own resolution process; a counselor feeling stuck in working with your clients who are trying to resolve their past trauma; or the loved one of either—my prayer for you is that within this book you will find HOPE. Not hope for salvation, because that only comes from Jesus Christ, but hope for transformation. Hope that you don't have to live with all of this pain anymore. The pain can go away, for good.

Chapter One: Introducing Etiotropic Trauma Management and Trauma Resolution Therapy

"Etiotropic Trauma Management"—pronounced "eat-e-o-tro-pic"—comes from the root word etiology. Etiology refers to the source or cause of a disease or problem. *This* trauma management system is etiotropic in that it focuses all efforts on identifying, addressing and resolving trauma at its *source*. You could say we go to the root of the problem. This is the opposite of most other counseling methods which tend to be Nosotropic. Nosotropic approaches focus on reducing the symptoms of the trauma.

ETM is a theoretical model—a plan based on a theory—which provides strategies and implementation procedures for addressing all types of psychological trauma and its effects on individuals, families, relationships, communities and organizations. ETM was originally titled "Integrated Trauma Management System" by its developers Jesse Collins and Nancy Carson in the early 1980's. They changed the name in the mid 1990's to make it more distinctive from other trauma management systems. ETM is very different from all the others. ETM is the only method that focuses strictly on resolving the trauma at the *source*.

The application or treatment part of ETM theory is called *Trauma Resolution Therapy*. You can read more about the history and development of the ETM Model in Jesse Collins' book *The Integrated Trauma Management*

Denice Adcock Colson

System, available through the ETM Training Workshop. The history is also available on line at www.Etiotropic.org.

What Makes ETM Different?

ETM is the only treatment approach which focuses exclusively on resolving the trauma at the source rather than managing the symptoms. In fact, ETM goes as far as preventing attempts to change symptoms. Survivors are directly asked *not* to try to change symptoms until they have completed all five phases of the treatment process. (The only exceptions are the consumption of alcohol, illegal drugs and sedating prescription medications as well as suicide and self-mutilating behavior or physical violence against others.) This is not reverse psychology or a paradoxical intervention.

The structure of Trauma Resolution Therapy (TRT) is also designed to preclude participants from attempting to focus on or change their symptoms. I want to emphasize "attempt" here because, even though we are not focusing on changing symptoms, the symptoms are nevertheless eradicated when a person completes all five phases of TRT.

It is our belief that trauma survivors *need* their symptoms. Where there is etiology, there are going to be symptoms. In the same manner, where there are live roots, a plant will grow. Symptoms and etiology are forever linked in a paradoxical relationship. When you focus on the symptoms without first resolving the trauma, it can reinforce the symptoms and even create new symptoms and thus more damage. Prior to using ETM/TRT, I became mired in this paradox numerous times with clients. A specific example of this was the whole "Tough Love" movement. In this intervention parents were directed by their therapists to turn their teenagers out on the street if they refused to stop using drugs and alcohol and start following the rules. I told several parents to do this and became frustrated when they not only could not do it, but continued to enable their teens' substance abuse. Eventually they would realize that I could not help them and leave feeling hopeless. I would in turn assume that they did not want to stop enabling their child for some secret reason. Looking back now, I can see how absurd this was. I did not realize that I was putting the blame for the trauma they were experiencing (teen's substance abuse) back onto them. By asking them to do something that went against their own values and beliefs, I was creating more trauma (etiology) for them. By putting them in the position where they had to disappoint their counselor, I was also creating more etiology for them.

It is not that focusing on changing symptoms never seems to work. Quite the contrary. People seem to be able to make progress in changing some symptoms and that makes them feel successful. Counselors and theorists then think that all symptoms should be able to change given the right motivation. However, many symptoms seem to keep people stuck. Sometimes people just "swap" symptoms. They swap an obviously self-destructive behavior for a not so-obviously self-destructive behavior, and that looks better to everyone. Clients and counselors alike, however, become frustrated with this cycle. Worse yet, it leads to a sense of hopelessness. Eventually the client gives up, believing that he has a spiritual or character disorder that prevents him from ever being able to get past the trauma in his life. Therapists also become cynical and begin to doubt the possibility of real and complete healing and hope to just teach their clients to cope.

This is the paradox of focusing on changing symptoms before the trauma is resolved. Not only does it not work but also more etiology is created. When more etiology is created, more symptoms develop. When more symptoms develop, more damage is done to the person and to those around him or her. You see, typical psychotherapy has gradually moved toward the "medical model." This says that the symptoms are the problem. Since they cannot cure the disease, they treat the symptoms. ETM counselors believe that the trauma's *existence in memory* is the problem and the symptoms are the *natural* effects of the traumatic event.

So, what is the "source" or the "etiology" of trauma? According to ETM theory, the etiology or source of ongoing trauma is the *continuous contradiction of existential identity*. Existential identity refers to our basic personal identities, which are made up of the sum of our values, beliefs, image and reality. Our values are anything and everything we deem as valuable, such as peace, happiness, love, our bodies, our health, etc. Our beliefs include everything that we believe about ourselves and our world, such as, "I believe my husband should show me love and respect," or "I believe marriage should be forever." Image involves self-image as well as our image of others. Reality involves the integration of our values, beliefs and image with what we see, hear and experience.

ETM also theorizes that the continuous contradiction of existential identity is not just *psychological*, but that it actually has a *physiological* location in the brain. We believe that actual neurons in the brain are changed as a result of trauma. New memory patterns are developed which override pre-trauma memory patterns. In other words, originally held beliefs which are stored in the brain in the form of patterns of neurons are extinguished by newer and stronger patterns of neurons developed as a result of the trauma. These changes occur in the part of the brain that supports memory. It is as if the trauma were recorded in the "present tense" and remains this way until the etiology is reversed. Recent research supports the theory that Post-Traumatic Stress Disorder is a brain-based issue. The debate continues as to which part of the brain is specifically affected. There are several books and articles which discuss this in more technical terms than we will be using in this work. If you want to read more about brain research, be sure to check out the Bibliography on line at www.Etiotropic.org.

Differences between TRT and Other Helping Relationships

TRT is considered to be a "structured Psychodynamic" approach to resolving trauma. "Structured" refers to the fact that TRT utilizes a step-by-step, five-phase process which is designed to resolve the trauma. The purpose of the structure is to keep the focus of the therapy on the address of the etiology of the trauma until that address is fully completed and the etiology is fully reversed. "Psychodynamic" refers to a form of therapy which is primarily concerned with the individual's internal experiences. In recent years, many therapists have abandoned psychodynamic techniques because they tend to produce an overwhelming amount of information and emotion. The client and the therapist both tend to become overwhelmed and abandon the treatment. This has led to the idea of "re-traumatization." The belief is that by having the client "relive" the traumatic experience and all of the emotions attached, you are literally traumatizing the client again. This comes from the belief that the symptoms *are* the source of the problem or the trauma. TRT minimizes or prevents this overwhelming experience from happening by applying a very secure structure. Also, the view of symptoms in TRT is different than in behavioral techniques. Avoiding the memory of the trauma is not only impossible but also prevents the resolution of the trauma.

As I said before, ETM theory states that etiology causes symptoms and that etiology and symptoms have a cause and effect relationship. In other words, when there is etiology there will and must be symptoms. In ETM/TRT theory the term for symptoms is changed to "survival responses," personifying their normal and natural purpose in helping the person to survive. Symptoms must remain until the etiology is fully reversed. The symptoms serve to distract the survivor, keeping the focus off the repressed pain and loss.

Etiology reversal or trauma resolution means that the existential identity (values, beliefs, images and reality) is reconstituted to its pre-trauma existence but within the context of the current period. In other words, the pre-event values, beliefs, images and reality are restored but within the current context of time, age, level of maturity and life situation. This happens not only on a psychological level but also on a physiological level. It is our hypothesis that the nerve pathways and memory systems are literally restored to pre-event configurations.

Treatment of trauma-related issues, including Post-Traumatic Stress Disorder and Acute Stress Reaction, occur on a continuum. Where etiology focused treatment occurs at one end, nosotropic approaches represent the other end or exact opposite. Nosotropic methods focus either on symptom reduction or on both etiology and symptom reduction. For example, behaviorism focuses strictly on reducing the negative symptoms, while cognitive behavioral and non-structured psychodynamic approaches focus on both the etiology and the reduction of symptoms. TRT, on the other hand, focuses only on etiology reversal and even precludes attempts to change or reduce symptoms until the etiology is fully reversed. Precluding "attempts" to change symptoms is the most significant difference between TRT/ETM and other theories and methodologies. "Attempts" is emphasized because, although there are no *attempts* to alter symptoms, they nevertheless are eradicated following the complete reversal of the etiology. When the etiology is gone, the symptoms, or survival responses, are no longer needed and end on their own. My experience has been that clients will stop in the process at some point and ask themselves, "When did I stop doing that? I don't remember trying to change it, and I don't remember when it stopped." For example, "When did I stop letting people walk all over me?" or "When did I stop eating to deal with my guilt?" or "When did I stop thinking about suicide all the time?" It is an amazing phenomenon to watch and even more amazing to experience.

Specific Differences between TRT/ETM and Other Helping Models

Unstructured Psychodynamic approaches include Client-Centered therapy and traditional Grief therapy. Using these approaches, a counselor encourages a person to identify, experience, and express emotions. They may also help the trauma victim identify the significance of the trauma in his or her life. While these approaches are very similar to TRT, they are also different in some very significant ways.

1. Most Client-Centered and Psychodynamic approaches are unstructured, allowing the client to set the pace and topic of the day. TRT is very structured, planning every step of the therapeutic process for the individual.

2. Non-structured approaches encourage the identification of any emotional pain and loss, as they become available. Sometimes that emotion may be related to the trauma-causing event in question, but sometimes it may be related to something else. For example, a client was in the process of completing the five-phase TRT process on her husband's recent physical and verbal abuse. While listening to another group member read, she identified feelings related to past sexual abuse. A non-structured approach would encourage her to focus on the new feelings, experience them, process them and, thereby, switch the focus to the sexual abuse. TRT's structure kept her focused on the feelings related to her husband's abuse until she completed all five phases, then focused on the sexual abuse. An unstructured approach leads to diversion, confusion, and the experience of being emotionally overwhelmed. The structure of TRT prevents both diversion and the experience of being emotionally overwhelmed. It replaces confusion with clarity and uncertainty with certitude.

3. A non-structured approach leaves it up to the client to designate the completion of therapy based on how he or she feels. When resolving trauma, feelings are very labile, and identifying when the resolution is complete from an internal vantage point is impossible. The structure of TRT gives you an end. The approach is so thorough that, if you follow the directions, when you complete the fifth phase, you are *done*. The client is not left to question, "Have I resolved that or not?" He or she can know with certainty that it is completed.

Behavioral Therapy, or Cognitive-Behavioral Therapy, helps the trauma victim become more aware of his or her behavior and belief systems. The individual is then coached on how to change his or her unwanted behavior to adopt more successful coping mechanisms. There are many adaptations of this model. Some are Rational Emotive Therapy, Reality

Therapy, "Positive Thinking" therapies, and Behavior Therapy that utilizes techniques such as Systematic Desensitization and Classical Conditioning. All focus on the trauma victim's response to the trauma and to changing either the coping mechanisms or changing the way the person thinks about the trauma and themselves.

These techniques are very useful when correctly applied to the appropriate person or after trauma has been resolved. They can help people learn more appropriate ways of dealing with life and how to be more successful. Being a great believer in Rational Emotive Therapy, I used this approach with my trauma victims for years. I taught *The Search for Significance*, by Robert S. McGee, for several years. His approach is a Biblically based Cognitive-Behavioral model. Identify the "irrational" beliefs (or lies) and replace them with Biblical truths. I also used "Inner Healing," which is extremely similar to the current "Theophostic Therapy." Using visualization "controlled" by the Holy Spirit, you enter the memory, identify the "lies of Satan" and allow the Holy Spirit to replace them with God's truth. This is just another way, however, albeit strongly spiritual in focus, of cognitive restructuring. My personal experience was that for some people it worked, at least temporarily. They experienced great emotional release and learned their true value in the eyes of God. Others became increasingly frustrated and filled with guilt. The pattern I saw with Rational Emotive Therapy was, if trauma were involved, it would help the victim adjust to society more appropriately but would not resolve the hurt from the past. I now believe that all of these techniques worked to repress the trauma even further into the unconscious, shifting the focus to the individuals themselves and how they coped with the aftermath. I feel bad because, I believe for most of these people, the effects of the trauma probably came back up at a later time, and they would not necessarily associate the symptoms with the trauma since that had been "addressed" in past therapy. That would make the next therapist's job more difficult if he wanted to focus on resolving trauma, rather than managing it. Clinically, the differences between Cognitive Behavioral Therapy approaches and TRT include:

1. While Cognitive-Behavioral Therapies focus on behavior and changing the behavior, TRT's focus is on resolving the internally retained trauma. It is the philosophy of TRT that once the trauma is resolved, the individual will experience a change in his or her behavior on his/her own, even subconsciously, without advice from the counselor.

2. While Cognitive-Behavioral Therapy would view the trauma-initiated thoughts and behaviors of the trauma victim as "a behavioral disorder," or as "maladaptive," or even as "character defects," TRT believes that these new thoughts and behaviors are a *natural consequence* of the trauma.

Self-help groups come in many flavors. The goal of most self-help groups is to change your behavior, to make you a more responsible person, or to help you make more appropriate choices. While TRT is most often applied in a group setting, ***TRT is not a self-help program.***

1. TRT stresses the resolution of the trauma, not changing your behavior or personality.

2. TRT views the trauma-induced behavior and thoughts as *survival responses* which serve to protect the person from both the internally retained trauma and the possibility of future trauma experiences. (See Chapter Four entitled <u>Survival Responses</u> for more information.) Therefore, changing these protective behaviors before resolving the trauma would force the retained trauma to develop new survival responses.

3. TRT theory believes that, due to the way the trauma is retained in the unconscious and provides for its own protection, it is *impossible* for a trauma victim to learn to resolve trauma on his or her own. Someone from outside of the trauma victim *must* assist the person in moving through resolution. This person does not have to be a TRT trained therapist, but there are certain requirements for resolving trauma. If those are present in the person's life, he or she may resolve the trauma naturally, or as God has designed us to do. (See Chapter Two entitled <u>Understanding the Influence Trauma Has Had on Your Life</u> for more information.)

Systems Theory, which is used in most marriage and family therapy, approaches all individuals as though they are a part of a system. This theory focuses on making shifts in the system in order to bring balance and help everyone to get their needs met. While one systemic theory views the family which is adapting to trauma as "dysfunctional," TRT views the same family as "functional." TRT believes that the family is doing exactly what any other family would do in the face of trauma, such as an alcoholic parent or child, a physically abusive or sexually abusive parent or child. Again, Systems Theory would focus on changing the effects of the trauma, i.e., the boundary erosion and relationship fusion, seeing this as the *cause* of the dysfunction. TRT again focuses on resolving the trauma within the individual, which in turn restores management controls to the family and ends the boundary erosion and relationship fusion.

A therapist, trained in the correct use of Trauma Resolution Therapy, uses this model because it works. Their clients resolve their trauma and refer their friends and family. During my many years of experience with TRT, I have found it to be extremely helpful for a variety of trauma victims. TRT is not appropriate for *every* trauma victim, based not on the *type* of trauma, but on potential interfering factors. As you read the following chapters, I hope that you will make an informed choice about your involvement with TRT, either as a participant, a provider, or both.

Integrating Christian Faith with Trauma Resolution Therapy

The reality of my Christianity permeates my entire life. I cannot separate my Christian values and beliefs from my ministry in counseling. My approach to the use of *any* counseling technique is from a framework of Biblical principles. Although Trauma Resolution Therapy itself was not designed to be spiritual in nature, there is nothing in it that is contradictory to Scripture. The basic difference between Christian and non-Christian counseling is the focus. In non-Christian counseling, the focus is on *self-* actualization. In Christian counseling, the focus is on *God*-actualization. Self-actualization means that the self is fulfilled, that you be all you can be, get all you can get, do all you can do. God-actualization means that you become all God intends for you to be, which is Christ-like. The overriding goal of all Christian counseling should be to become more like Christ, to exude more of His character.

Etiotropic Trauma Management is based on the idea that we must address the root of the problem rather than treating the symptoms. We also need structure and assistance from someone else so that we are not deceived or confused by our own damaged brains. The process of Trauma Resolution Therapy is a tool that God can use to bring healing in individuals and families. Meeting together, comforting each other, confessing our sins to one another, affirming each other, and showing unconditional love to each other—these are all Biblical concepts. My experience in working with un-churched people has been that they develop a spiritual hunger as they resolve the trauma. They have been in so much pain that they may have overlooked that hole which only a relationship with their Creator can fill.

Denice Adcock Colson

The parable Jesus tells about the farmer going out to plant seed is one of my favorites. Some seed fell on rocky ground and took root, but the roots were shallow and the seed burned up in the sun. Some fell on soil with a lot of weeds. They grew up but the weeds choked them out. The weeds, Jesus explained, are the cares of the world. As I see it, using TRT to help people resolve trauma makes us gardeners, digging out rocks, pulling up weeds and preparing the soil so that the seed can grow deep roots and healthy fruit.

Chapter Two: Understanding The Influence Trauma Has Had On Your Life

In most cases, trauma is a sudden, invasive, externally initiated event. The severity of all traumas is equalized in the ETM model. There are no degrees of severity making one type worse than another. All types of trauma are equally severe. Remember that we are focusing on the source of the trauma. The source or etiology of trauma--ALL traumas--is torn-apart identity. A person's identity is either torn apart or not. There may be degrees of torn-apartness, but any degree of torn identity is still painful. What has torn my identity apart may not tear your identity apart. Trauma includes, but is not limited to, the following: chemical dependency, codependency (those in relationships with chemically dependent people), crime (sexual, physical assault), incest, disease (cancer, AIDS, etc.), family violence, child abuse, combat, accidents, natural catastrophes, and crisis management employment (EMT's, police officers, doctors, nurses, counselors, etc....). I have also applied TRT to verbal abuse—which is usually associated with drug addiction or mental illness, but not always—unwanted divorce, affairs, ng or spending addiction and miscarriage.[1]

most cases" trauma is externally initiated. In the case ction, spending addiction, sexual addiction, and other rs, the "toxic" behavior is indeed performed by the han by someone else. It is, however, considered to be outside the survivor, since it is behavior generated by the addiction rather than by the survivor's own existential identity. This will make more sense as we review the patterns of trauma and will be discussed in more depth as we talk about addiction as trauma for the addict.

Now let us review in more depth the four patterns of trauma. Remember that these patterns fall under two categories, the Initial Effects of Trauma, and the Life-Long Effects of Trauma.

Patterns of Trauma

Initial Effects

Pattern 1: An extraordinary event threatens or disrupts the ongoing status of the psychological management system; the threat or disruption <u>contradicts existential identity</u>. In other words, one's experience of the initial event contradicts one's values, beliefs, image and reality.

- **VALUES** are anything you consider to be important. You can value an idea, a thing, a person, a philosophy, a relationship, a lifestyle, etc.

- **BELIEFS** are your opinions and convictions.

- **IMAGE** is the representation of a specific person. In TRT "image" usually refers to self-image or the image of someone loved.

- **REALITY** is the sum of conscious and unconscious perception as that perception interacts with values, beliefs and image. In TRT "reality" usually relates to the perception of physical reality.

Pattern 2: Loss and emotion resulting from the contradictions are maintained in memory, conscious and unconscious. Losses include tangibles and intangibles such as self-esteem, self-respect, respect for the other person, innocence, sense of safety, femininity, masculinity, childhood, etc. These losses—along with the emotions accompanying them—are then repressed.

Life-Long Effects

Pattern 3: Repressed loss and emotion in Pattern 2 produce survival responses; they also can and do <u>contradict existential identity.</u> Survival responses are new thoughts, behaviors and perceptions that, although helpful at the time, may also contradict one's values, beliefs, image and reality.

Pattern 4: The survival response-induced contradictions (pattern 3) produce more loss and emotion which is also maintained in memory, both conscious and unconscious (repressed).

Consider the following real life example: Anna married Jim when she was in her late twenties. They met in a Bible-study. Everyone thought they were the perfect couple. Out of spiritual conviction, they decided not to have sex until they were married. Though Anna was very excited about making love to Jim, on their wedding night she was exhausted. She suggested to Jim that they cuddle and hold each other until they fell asleep then make love the next morning. Jim told her that he was very disappointed in her and insisted that she do her wifely duty and have sex with him immediately. She pleaded that she would enjoy their first intimate experience much more when she was rested. Jim told her that to be a good wife she must have sex when her husband wanted it and that she would get used to it and enjoy it—after all, other women did. Fearing her husband's rejection, Anna did not fight as he, without foreplay, had intercourse with her. Instead, she cried silently as he reached orgasm. When he finished, he was angry that she had gotten blood on him and the sheets. He went into the bathroom and again expressed how disappointed he was in her. When he returned, she cuddled close to him and put her arm around him seeking comfort. He pushed her away saying, "I'm sleepy, leave me alone." As he went to sleep, she crept silently into the bathroom and sat on the floor and cried.

Throughout this book I will refer to Anna (not her real name) who experienced several more years of severe sexual, physical and verbal abuse. This, however, was her first experience of abuse. Prior to the wedding night, her fiancée had been the model of a Christian gentleman. Although he had some negative behavior in his past, he claimed to have developed a relationship with Jesus Christ and, to all appearances, had truly changed. He gave no clue as to his true character prior to the wedding. Let us identify the patterns in this incident.

Initial Effects

Pattern 1: Jim's thoughtless, insulting attitude and statements about Anna's tiredness, his insistence that they have sex against her wishes, his utter disregard for her sexual satisfaction, and his cold brush off after he "finished" all contradicted Anna's personal values, her beliefs about relationships, marriage and sex, her image of her new husband and her life reality. Anna believed her husband should be tender, caring, and understanding. She believed he should consider her physical well-being and that lovemaking should be a mutual decision. She believed her wedding night should be special and memorable for its closeness and emotional and spiritual bonding. She believed her husband was a man of character, that he loved her more than he loved himself. She believed she was in a committed, God-centered marriage which would be mutually satisfying and last until they died.

Pattern 2: The contradictions resulting from Anna's experience of her husband's abusive behavior resulted in loss. Anna lost self-esteem, trust, and respect for her husband and for herself, a precious and beautiful experience, intimacy, closeness and more. When she sought comfort from her husband for these losses, he shut down communication with her. Since there was no way to reconcile her losses, they—along with the emotions accompanying them—were repressed into her unconscious.

Life-Long Effects

Pattern 3: Anna's repressed losses fostered survival responses in her. She withdrew from her husband emotionally and put on a smile around him, not showing her true feelings. The next day she acted like nothing happened. She pushed herself to have sex whenever he wanted and did not complain if she was uncomfortable. She lied to her friends and family about how wonderful the honeymoon was. All of these behaviors contradicted Anna's beliefs about how she should behave. She believed she should be open and honest with her husband, that she should be emotionally vulnerable to him, and that she should be honest with her friends and family.

Pattern 4: Anna's experience of her own survival responses contradicting her values, beliefs, image and reality resulted in more loss. She lost more self-esteem, self-respect, self-confidence, intimacy with her husband and family and friends. With no way to reconcile her additional losses, these—

along with the emotions accompanying them—were also repressed into her unconscious.

Back up a moment and pretend that the next day Jim was truly repentant and said to Anna, "I'm very sorry about last night. I was wrong. Please forgive me." Anna would have continued to feel hurt and would have still experienced some losses, but they would not have been repressed. As a couple, they could process the experience and go on with their lives. True repentance means that you turn away from the sin and you do not do it again.

Let us consider an example of a single-episode trauma. Mark was in his early forties and worked at a large refining plant. One day at work the warning signals went off and he heard an explosion. He ran, with his fellow employees, out of the plant and into a field. He stopped to help a fellow employee who had injured her leg. Smoke was everywhere. People were screaming and running. He began to run toward a ravine when another large blast occurred. It shook his body and left a ringing sound in his ears. He stumbled and fell. Feeling a sharp pain in his left hand, he lay there dazed and confused. Finally a friend stopped and helped him up. They continued until they were outside the fence. He heard sirens now heading towards them, but he felt disoriented and numb. Later, he found out that two people had been killed in the explosion.

Initial Effects

Pattern 1: The explosion, the personal injury, and the deaths of fellow employees all contradicted Mark's personal beliefs, values, and reality. He believed he was safe working in the administration building of the refinery. He valued his job and his fellow employees. He believed this would never happen to him. He felt shocked, terrified, and horrified.

Pattern 2: The contradictions between Mark's values, beliefs, image and reality resulted in losses of confidence, trust, security, safety, self-reliance, respect for his job, and the lives of two co-workers. These losses were repressed.

Life-Long Effects

Pattern 3: The repressed loss which originated from the initial trauma fostered survival responses. Mark was terrified to return to work. He became very sensitive to sudden or loud noises and startled easily. He withdrew from his family and friends and found himself becoming increasingly depressed and anxious. He began taking a lot of prescribed medication. These survival responses also contradicted Mark's values, beliefs, image and reality. He believed he should be able to handle anything. He believed he should always be there for his wife and children. He believed depression was a sign of weakness and medication was for those who could not take care of themselves.

Pattern 4: Mark developed more loss. He lost self-esteem, self-confidence, closeness with his children, intimacy with his wife. He lost his excellent health, his drive and his ambition. These losses were also repressed.

The effects of trauma develop with the *first* experience, whether or not more incidents occur. With one episode of trauma there will be multiple losses and may be multiple survival responses. Even though "it only happened once," if it is trauma, it still influences you. Many people minimize the effect of abuse because "it was only fondling," or "it only happened once." There *are* more losses experienced when abuse occurs more than once, or when the abuse is more intense. Nevertheless, while the trauma on the outside may be *different*, the *same* pattern develops internally for all traumas.

The Pre-Trauma Personal Identity of the Individual

Carson and Collins refer to the Personal Identity of an individual as being composed of the Existential Component and the Operational Component. The *Existential component (EC)* of personal identity consists of your values, beliefs, image and reality. The term "existential" is intended to emphasize that these attitudes exist as a basic fact of your psychological makeup. It also refers to the fact that these attitudes, however strongly held they might be, are *passive* as opposed to *active* oriented aspects of identity. In other words, this is the foundation and framework on which everything else about the person is built. This is the "being" part of one's personal identity, as opposed to the "doing." Carson and Collins use the image of a piece of fabric, with its tightly woven threads, to illustrate the Existential Component of personal identity. The closeness of the threads represents how closely a person's values, beliefs, image and reality are associated with each other.[2]

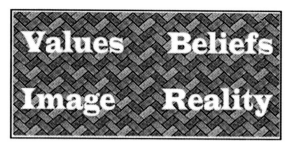

Figure 1: Existential Componant of Personal Identity

Some examples of values, beliefs, image and reality used by clients when completing Phase Two of TRT include:

- Christmas should be a happy time.
- Mothers should not get drunk.
- Husbands should not embarrass their wives in public.
- You should not drive when drunk.
- Fathers should show respect for their wives.
- Life is worth living.
- Suicide is wrong.
- I should not use illegal drugs.
- I saw my father as a role model.
- My boundaries should be respected.

The *Operational Component* of personal Identity is the "doing" part. There are two aspects of the Operational component. First are the "natural attributes," of which there are two kinds: the Rational/Cognitive attributes and the Experiential attributes. Many of the Operational Component's activities take place in the unconscious mind.

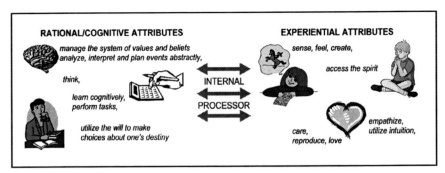

Figure 2: Two Types of Attributes in the Operational Component of Personal Identity

The Rational/Cognitive attributes can be characterized as the "head." This is the thinking and doing part of the identity. A person calls on these attributes when he is sizing up a situation about which he has to make a decision. When tasks like housecleaning or homework have to be completed, the choices are made out of this part of the identity.

The Experiential attributes can be characterized as the "heart." The touchy/feely attributes are accessed in relationships and in decision-making. That "gut instinct" about a new person you meet comes from these attributes of the identity.

The second aspect of the Operational Component is the "internal processor." This functions much like the central processing unit (CPU) of the computer on which I am typing. Without the CPU, the computer cannot assimilate the software with the hardware, nor can the software work together to assimilate the information I am putting into it. There are two interactive elements of the internal processor:

1. It controls the interaction between the natural attributes and values, beliefs, image and reality.

2. It controls the interaction between the natural attributes themselves.

Stop Treating Symptoms and Start Resolving Trauma!

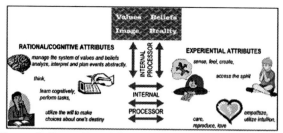

Figure 3: Operational Component of Personal Identity

In other words, prior to the occurrence of any trauma, while you are "doing" you are in touch with your "being," who you are as a person. You think and feel in line with your own personal values, beliefs, image and reality. Also when you are thinking, completing tasks, making choices about your life, you are feeling, you are in touch with your intuition and with your spirituality. As a whole, the aspects of your identity are well integrated. Generally, the Operational Component of Personal Identity makes choices about life, interacts with others, manages life's ups and downs, and protects you from harm by making wise choices which take in all aspects of the situation.

The Post-Trauma Personal Identity of the Individual

When a person experiences trauma, it simultaneously affects both the Existential Component and the Operational Component of one's Personal Identity. Let us talk about the Existential Component first.

Post-Trauma Existential Component of Personal Identity

When the traumatic event occurs, it contradicts your values, beliefs, image and reality. The "fabric" of your Existential Identity is "torn."

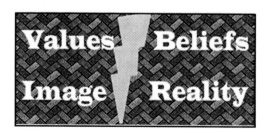

Figure 4: Post-Trauma Existential Identity

In other words, your fixed values, beliefs, image, and reality are no longer continuous. When this occurs, you experience losses.

There are eleven basic emotions that accompany a loss. They are shock, confusion, disbelief, fear, pity, shame, anger, hurt, depression, guilt and sadness. Collins and Carson diagram this as a "loss chain"—a thread with shock at one end, loss at the other end, and all of the other emotions in between.

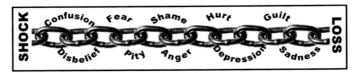

Figure 5: A Single Loss Chain

In one incident of trauma, many losses occur simultaneously. For example, when a boy is sexually abused by his uncle, he loses trust, innocence, safety, childhood, self-esteem and more, all at once. Each of these losses forms its own "loss chain."[3]

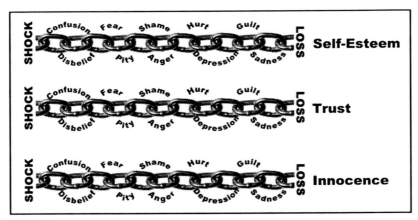

Figure 6: Multiple Loss Chains Line Up With Each Other

With the passing of time, it is as if the loss chains line up with each other. Confusion is lined up with confusion, anger with anger, loss with loss, etc. As more losses occur and more loss chains develop, they begin to move closer together, blurring their boundaries. It becomes difficult to distinguish one loss chain from another.

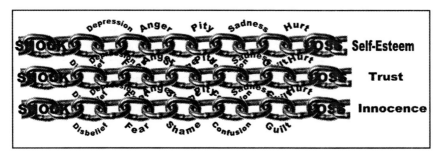

Figure 7: Loss Chains Become More Compressed.

Eventually, with the passing of time, they become *compressed*. Much like if you took a very hot iron and used it on a piece of fabric for an extended period of time, the fabric would scorch and the threads would become very tightly bonded together. As the loss chains become compressed, they become increasingly indistinguishable. One emotion fuses with another emotion and another and another. Now you have the formation of "streams of emotion."

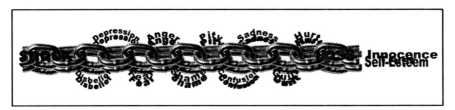

Figure 8: Compressed Loss Chains.

For example, all of the angers from all of the losses become tied together, much like a string of Christmas tree lights. When you plug it in, they all light up. The phenomenon of "acceleration"[4] occurs. When the person feels anger in the present, it attaches itself to all of the other repressed angers and pulls them all up. Thus, anger accelerates into rage. The person may be aware of overreacting to the situation, but he or she is caught up in the rush of emotion, much like a stick is caught in the rushing current of a river heading over a waterfall. Others around the person are also confused and may accuse the person of being too "dramatic" or of overreacting. All of the basic emotions which accompany loss and grief can succumb to the same acceleration phenomenon. Disbelief can accelerate into disorientation, confusion into chaos, fear into paranoia, shame into humiliation, depression into incapacitation, hurt into a deep wound. Sadness becomes so overwhelming it is no longer identifiable and guilt becomes chronic. Loss accelerates into catastrophic grief.

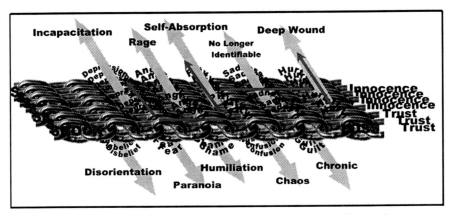

Figure 9: Streams of Emotion Cause Acceleration and Expansion.

Another phenomenon occurs which Collins and Carson call "expansion."[5] Not only are the emotions compressed vertically, but also horizontally. Thus, an emotional response can travel not only the length of a stream of emotion, but it can also travel from one stream to another. For example, a person may start out with fear which accelerates into paranoia, expand to hurt which accelerates to a deep wound, and then expand to anger, which accelerates to rage. This makes the emotional experience of the victim much more complex and difficult to understand or reconcile. At this point the person is totally overwhelmed with his or her emotional experience and may even question his or her own sanity. Since this emotional experience is so intensely painful subconsciously, or consciously, the trauma survivor makes the decision to avoid his or her emotions as much as possible.

This maze of emotional circuitry and loss now joins together in one solid loss formation. Shock, the most powerful and protective emotion of them all surrounds the loss formation to protect the person from recognizing the repressed maze of emotional pain and loss. Shock also blocks conscious awareness of the damage done to the Existential Identity, as well as the disintegrating values, beliefs, image and reality.

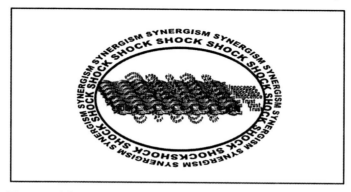

Figure 10: Maze of Emotional Ciruitry and Loss.

As this "maze" remains in the unconscious, it eventually begins to provide for its own existence by adding more protective components. Unit cohesiveness develops into "synergism." According to the American Heritage Dictionary, synergism refers to "the action of two or more substances, organs, or organisms to achieve an effect of which each is individually incapable."[6] In other words, the identity of each loss chain is given over to the power of the whole. Consider a football team whose players are individually very powerful. The more they become interrelated and work together, the more powerful they become. Their unit strength, or teamwork, is synergism.

At this point, survival responses begin to develop. Their purpose initially is to help the individual to live through the traumatic experience. As time goes by, however, their purpose is expanded to also help keep the focus off the internal pain and create a false sense of being in control. To be fair, these last two purposes are also seen by the survivor as necessary to survival. What we call survival responses, other theorists' call symptoms and defense mechanisms. These may be new behaviors, thoughts, perceptions, or attitudes which serve to help the psyche—or identity—survive through the trauma. Some examples of survival responses listed by clients in their Phase Three writings include:

- I doubted my ability to be a good wife.
- I tried to anticipate what you wanted.
- I blamed myself.
- I waited for you to change.

- I made excuses not to spend time with you.
- I thought I lacked faith, or God would have helped me.
- I slept on the floor to avoid you.
- I cried.
- I glared at you.
- I lied about the bruises.
- I thought I was stupid.
- I hated you.
- I laughed and made jokes about you.
- I became mean and controlling with my friends.
- I ate to feel better.

Unfortunately, many survival responses also contradict the individual's values, beliefs, image, and reality about themselves and how he or she should be acting. These contradictions, just as with the initial trauma, result in another tear in the Existential Identity of the person. Therefore—more loss is experienced, more loss chains form, more of the emotions which are associated with grief are experienced, and—the entire process is reproduced a second time. Now there are two rips in the Existential Identity, two emotional mazes, and two synergistic entities which join together to resist all attempts at resolving the repressed loss and emotion.

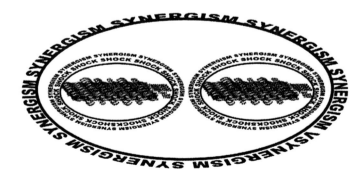

Figure 11: Two Mazes Joined Together With Synergism.

Post-Trauma Operational Component of Personal Identity

The Operational Component of the Personal Identity is also affected. First, the Internal Processor is interrupted. The flow of information between the Rational/Cognitive and the Experiential aspects is stopped so that the thinking and feeling are no longer working together. A woman may rationally know that she is making a poor decision, but her feelings are so strong that she moves in the wrong direction. Or, she may have a check in her spirit about doing something but ignore it because of the stronger rationale. The interaction between the Operational Component and the Existential component is also interrupted. So when the person is making decisions and managing his or her life, he or she is completely unaware of the damage that has been done to the values, beliefs, image and reality.

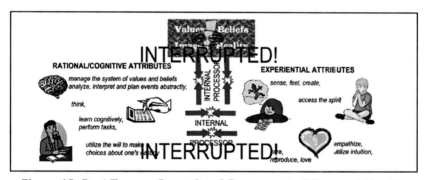

Figure 12: Post-Trauma Operational Component of Personal Identity

Thus, the person becomes divided. She is no longer accessing all of herself when making choices, learning, experiencing, or feeling. She may look back on decisions made during this time and ask, "What was I thinking?" People around her wonder why she cannot see things that are so obvious to them but are so invisible to the survivor. This is how people make such bad decisions about relationships after trauma. There are many books about women continuing to choose abusive or neglectful men with whom to get involved. It is not that they are *reinventing* the trauma experience or *causing* the men to turn bad because that is how they are comfortable. They truly *cannot* see the warning signs of a bad relationship, and someone's pointing it out to them rarely helps.

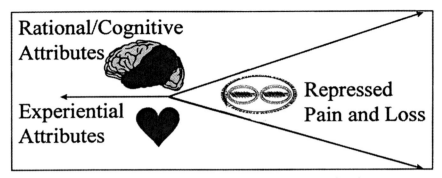

Figure 13: Summary of Divided Operational Identity.

In this divided state, the Operational Component compensates for the lack of integration by developing a special psychological apparatus which filters all information. Information from the environment, self or others passes through this filter and is altered in a way that makes assimilation of the information more tolerable to the individual.

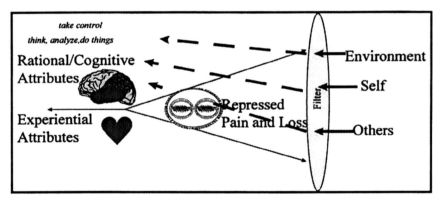

Figure 14: The Development of the Survivor.

This alteration is done by increasing reliance on the Rational/Cognitive attributes. The individual begins to try to take more control, use his or her willpower, *and do* something about it. As the individual's reliance on the Rational/Cognitive attributes increases, accessibility to the Experiential attributes decreases. For example, many survivors of sexual abuse read everything they can find about sexual abuse. They research and they study. They may even attend support groups and report what took place when they were traumatized, but all the while they become less and less connected to their feelings. Many survivors walk into my office and tell me horrible stories with straight faces and no tears. They tell me what is wrong with them and what they need to do to get over it, but they show no emotion about the abuse. On the other hand, they are emotionally out of control in many other areas of their lives. They are baffled as to why they can understand so much about their condition and yet nothing seems to change. This is a result of the divided state of the Operational Component of the identity.

With the continuing use of this process of screening, altering, and assimilating information with a rational/cognitive bias, the "filter" develops an identity of its own. Collins and Carson call this the "Survivor." [7]

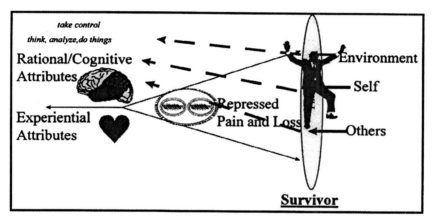

Figure 15: The Survivor Filters All Information.

With the inception of the Survivor, a paradox develops. The Survivor knows that buried in the unconscious there is emotional damage which is a danger to the person and that it is the responsibility of the Survivor to reconcile the damage. The unconscious aspects of the Survivor work toward achieving that goal and reconciling the damage. The conscious side of the Survivor recognizes its own protective qualities. It utilizes its ability to perform tasks and uses willpower to attempt to control situations. The Survivor begins to develop a *new* reality that denies the existence of the damage and takes over as the *actual Person*. The Survivor vows to protect the Person, using all of the resources it has available.

Consequently, the Survivor is in a constant tug-of-war with itself. On the one hand the unconscious aspect of the Survivor is attempting to get the trauma resolved. On the other hand the conscious aspect of the Survivor is attempting to keep the trauma and all of the emotional pain and damage repressed. This creates a great deal of tension in the individual. One week he or she seems keenly aware of the need to resolve this past trauma and reconcile its effects. The next week he does not think he needs to devote any time to focusing on the past—after all it does not affect him anyway. The longer the Survivor is in existence in the individual, the more control it has over the person's perception of reality, and the more the Survivor is identified as the Person. To illustrate this point, let us look at the saying, "Your mind is like an iceberg." An iceberg is a huge mountain of ice in an ocean. There is much more ice underneath the water than is showing above the water.

The ice above the water line represents the conscious mind, and the ice below the water represents the unconscious mind. The conscious aspect of the Survivor attempts to raise the water line, placing more information into the unconscious (below the water) and minimizing the information in the conscious mind (above the water).

The unconscious aspect of the Survivor attempts to lower the water line, exposing the information repressed in the unconscious mind.

The dilemma is, if the trauma is resolved, there will be no need for the Survivor, and it will cease to exist. So, in order for it to provide for its own existence, it must keep the trauma repressed. Thus, when victims of childhood trauma consider Trauma Resolution Therapy, a common concern is "Who am I?" Since the Survivors have existed for most of their lives, they are afraid of who they will be without them. They are afraid they may not be able to protect themselves from future hurt, pain, or trauma. On the other hand, if the trauma continues unresolved, the repressed pain and loss continue to remain in the unconscious, and the Survivor must continue to compensate for the divided state of the identity. More and more Survivor interactions must be initiated. As they contradict the person's values and beliefs, more pain and loss result. Either way the person goes, he or she seems to lose, and therefore he or she perceives himself or herself as stuck.

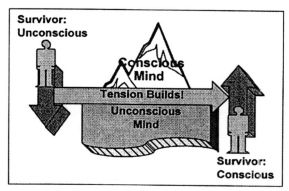

Figure 16: There Is A Constant Tug-Of-War Between the Conscious and Unconscious Aspects of the Survivor.

These new Survivor initiated interactions serve two *opposing* purposes. One is to resolve the trauma, and the other is to prevent the resolution of that same trauma. This pulling of the person in two opposite directions results in contradictory behaviors and thoughts. When looking at the behaviors and thoughts without considering the internal damage to the Existential Identity—and the subsequent breakdown of the internal processor—some of the behaviors may appear to be helpful or adaptive, and others harmful or maladaptive. In TRT these opposing behaviors are seen as a natural result of the trauma-causing event and are labeled as "Survival Responses."

Chapter Three: The Effect Of Trauma On Families and Other Relationships

Families are truly the backbones of our societies. The family is the system around which all other relationships are formed. When a family is influenced by trauma, it begins to fall apart. Even if the trauma is a secret, as is often the case with sexual abuse, *everyone* is touched. As relationship fusion takes its toll on the family, management of the family becomes ineffective. The management is the responsibility of the adults, or parents. This includes making plans, decisions, communication and coordinating general activities. This occurs even when the perpetrator is not one of the parents. For example, Mr. And Mrs. Smith came in for marriage counseling. In the process of an evaluation I learned that their 15 year old daughter, Ginny, was sneaking out at night, verbally abusing her mother, had been picked up for curfew violation and was generally rebellious and disrespectful. After interviewing Ginny, I learned that she was drinking beer and hard liquor, smoking cigarettes and pot, and had experimented with some other hallucinogenic drugs. Mr. and Mrs. Smith could not agree on how to discipline Ginny and were having great difficulties communicating and getting along at all. They could not see that Ginny was in the early stages of alcoholism and drug addiction. Using TRT phases, they began to see that the problem was Ginny's addiction and not them.

Families are systems. Many well-known family theorists and teachers use a mobile to illustrate this fact. They use a mobile just like the black and white animals on strings suspended over a baby's crib, only with a mother, father, and children at the end of each pole rather than clowns or bears.

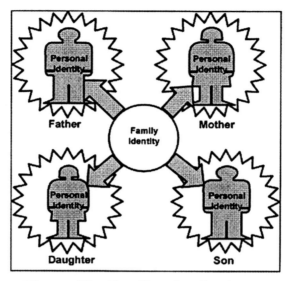

Figure 17: Families Are Systems.

When you move one family member, it affects the others. When a family is affected by ongoing trauma, say an alcoholic parent or a drug addicted child, everyone in the family, including extended family, is influenced. The members get caught up in the battle against the trauma's influences. As each incident occurs, non-trauma affected life is left behind and the family focuses on dealing with the internally retained trauma, as well as attempting to prevent the trauma from occurring again.

Let us look at the development of trauma in one family. Meet the Crenshaws. Bob Crenshaw is 36 and the father of the family. He works as a manager in an oil company. He has been drinking beer since he was 18 years old but has never been addicted. Mary is 33 years old and the mother of the family. She works part time from home as a computer programmer. She also manages the house and the children. She has been drinking beer off and on since she was 18 years old but has never been addicted. Sue Crenshaw is 14 years old and in the 9th grade. She has been an A/B student since she started school. John is 11 years old and in the 6th grade. He has been an A/B student since he started school. Neither has been in any significant trouble in school. Although it is unrealistic, for the sake of this example, the family has had no trauma or serious problems

Stop Treating Symptoms and Start Resolving Trauma!

of which to speak. Neither of the adults has any trauma in his or her background. For the sake of this example, we will make Bob, the father, the perpetrator of trauma in the family. The perpetrator could be anyone of the four, however.

First Incident

The family is at a restaurant with two other neighborhood families celebrating New Year's Eve. The kids are sitting together at a separate, but nearby table, while the adults are sitting men with men and women with women at their table. Bob had a couple of beers at home before coming to the restaurant and has had several more while at the restaurant. Mary notices that Bob seems to be laughing louder and louder. She hears a loud crash and turns to see her husband covered with spaghetti sauce and his plate on the floor. As she jumps up to help him he growls at her, "I can take care of myself, stupid!" He stands, very wobbly, and heads to the men's room. As everyone watches, he walks toward the door, showing a little bit of uncertainty in his steps.

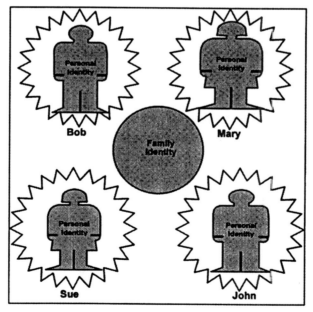

Figure 18: Crenshaw Family System Prior To Trauma.

In this first incident of trauma Bob has crossed that invisible line between social drinker and alcoholic. As he displays toxic behavior, the trauma affects him just as it does the rest of the family, and even the friends. First let us look at how the mother is affected. As Mary watches her husband she feels shocked, confused, anxious, embarrassed and angry. Her husband's drunken behavior contradicts her values, beliefs, image, and reality. She believes that he should not get drunk, especially not in front of their neighbors. She believes he should not call her names at home or in public. She believes he should act like a gentleman and be a role model for the children.

As Sue watches her father's behavior, she feels shocked, embarrassed, humiliated, scared and angry. Her father's drunken behavior also contradicts her values, beliefs, image and reality. She believes her father should be quiet and not draw attention to himself or to the family. She has never seen her father drunk before and believes that fathers should not get drunk.

As John watches his father's behavior, he also feels shocked, confused, embarrassed, and worried. His father's behavior also contradicts his values, beliefs, image and reality. He has never seen his father or anyone drunk before and believes that fathers should act normal and sane.

At this time we will not discuss Bob's experience of this episode, since he is the perpetrator. We will discuss it at length later on in the scenario.

The family unit's values and beliefs are also contradicted. The family rules are to be on your best behavior in public, do not call each other names, treat people with respect, and drinking until you are drunk is stupid.

When Bob's toxic behavior contradicts the family members' values and beliefs, they each experience losses. Mary loses respect for her husband, self respect, femininity, security, and intimacy with her husband. As she takes these losses to him in an attempt to reconcile them, she finds that he has shut her out. In order to protect himself, now that *he is an addict*, Bob has shut down his communication with those around him. When Mary is rebuffed, in order to protect herself, she must also shut down her communication system.

Because Mary has no place to reconcile her losses, rather than the losses remaining in her conscious, they are repressed in her personal identity. We will represent this repression with a √.

The children also experience losses and the shutting down of their communication systems. Sue experienced losses of self-esteem, confidence, security, femininity, and her father as a role model. John experienced losses of security, self-esteem, innocence, and a role model for how men behave. Since they have no place to deal with these losses, they are also repressed in their personal identities.

The repressed loss and emotion fosters the development of survival responses. Each family member develops his or her own set of new behaviors, beliefs and ideas which help at the time, but also contradict their values, beliefs, image, and reality. As a result of the first incident, Mary attempts to control her husband's behavior in subtle ways. She checks how much he drinks during the day. She tries to keep him from drinking when they go out. She also avoids her neighbors and lies to her parents about the incident. She minimizes the incident to the children saying, "Daddy just didn't feel well." These behaviors contradict Mary's own values and beliefs about how she believes she should be behaving. She believes that she should be honest, that she should not have to monitor her husband's behavior, and that she should socialize with her friends. As a result of these contradictions, Mary loses self-esteem, self-respect, and peace in her relationship with her husband, closeness with her parents and her children and much more. These losses are also repressed in her personal identity. As we diagram the effect of the trauma on the family members, these repressed losses will be represented with an **X**.

Sue begins to avoid going out with her parents, lying about eating at friends' houses, or manipulating friends to allow her to stay at their houses for dinner. She avoids extended contact with her father, even turning down shopping trips. She lies to her friends about her father's behavior and spends more time locked up in her room. These behaviors contradict Sue's values and beliefs about what she should be doing. She believes that she should tell the truth, that she should enjoy her family, and that she should spend time with her father, especially if getting new clothes is involved. Because of these contradictions, Sue loses self-esteem, closeness with her friends and family, new clothes, and much more. Sue's losses are also repressed in her personal identity.

John begins to worry about his father and to cling to him more. He starts to act younger than he is in an attempt to keep his father occupied with him. He gets in trouble at school for not listening and at home for talking "baby talk" and spilling things more often. These behaviors contradict

John's values and beliefs about what he should be doing. He believes that eleven years old is a more mature age and that he should be acting older. He believes that boys who act like babies are wimps. He believes that he should not get in trouble at school. John, therefore, loses self-esteem, friends, respect, his standing in school and more. His losses are also repressed.

As a whole, the family loses face in the community. They lose closeness with their neighbors and friends. Since they cannot communicate at this point to resolve the losses, they are repressed in the family identity. They develop, as a whole, survival responses. These include avoiding talking about the problem, pretending nothing happened, keeping secrets from people outside the family, and avoiding feelings. These behaviors contradict the family values and therefore cause more losses. These new losses are also repressed in the family identity.

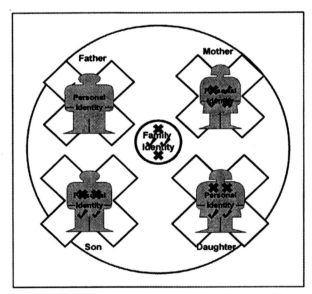

Figure 19: This Is How the Family Looks After One Incident of Trauma.

Second Incident

The next week Bob calls on Thursday afternoon and says he has to work late and will not be home in time for supper. Mary calls him around

6 pm but he does not answer his phone in his office. She calls his cell phone and he does not answer that either. She leaves a message in both places and waits for his call. At 7 pm she is worried. He still has not responded. She tries both his phones again and he still does not answer. She paces the floor, busies herself cleaning up after dinner and the kids, snaps at the kids and finally at 8 pm tries again, but still there is no answer. After she gets the kids in bed at 9 pm she calls Bob's mother and father to see if they have heard from him. "No," they reply, "But he's probably just really busy and doesn't want to be interrupted." Sensing that something is really wrong, Mary calls a friend who is an ER nurse and asks her how to check hospitals for new accident admissions. Her friend suggests she keep calling him on his cell phone while she calls the local emergency centers. At 11 pm her friend calls back to report that no one has had a Robert Crenshaw admitted to the hospital, but they did have one John Doe. Mary feels panicked wondering if this could be Bob. She hangs up and calls his cell phone one more time. This time Bob answers with, "What the hell do you want?!" Shocked and a little relieved Sue says, "Where have you been? I've been calling you all evening? Why didn't you answer your phone?" Twenty minutes later Bob walks through the front door, obviously drunk and very angry. He proceeds to yell at Mary, calling her names and insulting her. Finally he goes into the bedroom and slams the door. Shocked and confused, Mary sits in the living room crying. When she goes into the bedroom a little while later, Bob is asleep, and his clothes are all over the floor. The next morning he behaves as if nothing ever happened and so does Mary.

In this second incident of trauma, Bob's toxic behavior once again contradicts his family's values, beliefs, image and reality. Mary believes that her husband should be honest with her, should come home to his family rather than going out and getting drunk after work, and should never drive while drunk. She also believes that her husband should not yell at her, call her names or insult her. As a result of the contradictions, Mary experiences more losses. She loses respect for her husband, trust, family pride, confidence, security, self-esteem, and more. Because she cannot reconcile these losses, they are repressed.

Repressed loss and emotion fosters survival responses. Mary begins to quiz Bob in subtle ways on his whereabouts. She begins to check up on him at work by calling his secretary to find out where he is and when he leaves. She lies to her friend who is an ER nurse and her in-laws, saying that his phone died and he had forgotten to call home due to a frantic dead-line at work. She lies to the children, saying he just had to work late and was sorry for missing dinner with them. Since Mary's survival behaviors also contradict her values and beliefs about how she should be behaving, she experiences even more losses of self-confidence, self-esteem, closeness with friends and family, self-respect and more. These losses, accompanied by the normal grief emotions, are also repressed in the existential identity.

Even though the children were mostly unaware of the details of the incident, as a whole, the family experiences more loses of communication, trust, peace of mind, closeness and more. They also increasingly isolate themselves and withdraw from friends and family. The losses that result are repressed in the family identity.

Up until this point we have not addressed what is going on with Bob—the perpetrator of the trauma in our scenario. Do you think it was his intention to go to the New Year's Eve party, get drunk, humiliate his family, alienate his friends, and generally make a fool of himself? No, of course not. No one *plans* to become an alcoholic. He went to have fun. He drank to have fun. But, unknown to him, he crossed that invisible line between social drinker and alcoholic. His own toxic (drunk) behavior contradicted his own values and beliefs also. (In ETM we treat addiction and toxic under-the-influence-behavior as a perpetrator. For a full explanation of this please read the chapter on Addiction as Trauma for the Addict.) He believes that he should always conduct himself with dignity, and that he should not swear at his wife, especially in public. He believes that he should not get drunk around his children and humiliate them in front of their friends. These contradicted values and beliefs result in loss and the normal emotions which accompany loss. In order to avoid dealing with the loss and pain and to be able to continue drinking, he stops communicating. This does not mean he has stopped talking but that he is not *really* communicating. Now he is not only drinking alcohol but has also shut down his communication system, and his losses are also repressed.

As with everyone else, the repressed loss fosters survival responses for Bob. Bob pretended the incident never happened, but when confronted by his wife blamed his friend sitting across the table from him, blamed the waiter and blamed her for picking the restaurant. Other survival responses included denying the incident, pretending it never happened, minimizing it to himself and others, blaming his wife and her friends, and drinking more to help forget about it. These behaviors also contradict his values and beliefs about what he should be doing, although at this point to him his behavior is completely justified, and therefore he experiences more losses. He loses self-esteem, self-respect, and closeness with his family and friends, intimacy with his wife, self-confidence, and much more. These losses are also repressed in his personal identity.

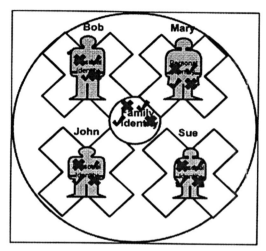

Figure 20: The Family After Two Incidents of Trauma.

Third Incident

A year has passed and several more incidents have occurred like the first two. The family even entered therapy in an attempt to help Sue, now 15, from failing in school. Bob's drinking has remained unaddressed, however. One Tuesday evening, Mary gets a call from a friend. She says that her husband saw Bob at a bar the previous week, he was with another woman, and they were both drinking pretty heavily. Mary is shocked! She calls Bob on his cell phone. He does not answer. She calls over and over again. Finally, Bob answers and says, "What the hell do you want! I'm busy here!" Mary can hear music and bar sounds in the background. She can tell he has been drinking by the way he is speaking. She asks him where he is and he says, "I'm trying to have a drink with a client. What do you want? Is it an emergency? What?" She tells him she thinks he is with another woman. He pauses, then starts laughing and says, "You're crazy! You need to see a psychiatrist!" He hangs up on her. Mary sits and cries in her room. The kids are in the family room playing on the computer and watching TV. Fifteen minutes later, she hears Bob come in the door. He starts cussing at the kids, screaming at them to go to bed. They try to argue but he starts pushing them and throwing things. Mary goes in to try to intervene and Bob starts yelling at her. The kids scream at him that they hate him and retreat to their rooms and slam their doors. Mary turns and stomps to her room and slams the door also. Bob follows swearing and yelling at her. He tries to open the door but it is locked. He starts banging on the door, yelling for her to open it. He starts kicking it and banging it, now in a rage, until he finally breaks it off its hinges and gets in. Mary is terrified! Bob grabs her by the shoulders, screaming and cussing and insulting her. He tells her that she ruined his deal and that she was obviously the one having an affair. He continues to shake her, then suddenly lets go of her. She backs up into the closet stunned, sits down against the wall and starts crying hysterically. Bob says, "You're pitiful!" then walks out the door and leaves the house and spends the night somewhere else.

Once again Bob's toxic behavior contradicts everyone's values and beliefs, including his own. They

1. experience more losses as a result of the contradictions;
2. repress the losses and emotions;
3. develop more survival responses which contradict their values and beliefs; and
4. experience more losses as a result of these contradictions, and the whole thing is repressed.

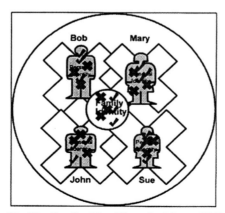

Figure 21: The Family After Three Incidents Of Trauma.

Stop Treating Symptoms and Start Resolving Trauma!

Without help from outside of the system, a family caught up in this degenerative spiral cannot stop itself. The family will fall apart. This may mean divorce, death, legal problems or some other tragic consequence. The family members will split up and go their separate ways, taking with them the internally retained affects of the trauma. Even though the trauma has ended, the survival responses *will* continue. As long as the trauma remains repressed in the subconscious, survival responses will continue and new responses will be developed. As the family members enter new relationships, they may be with perpetrators, trauma victims, or neither. The individuals they develop relationships with are a result of who they are around rather than an unconscious desire to return to revictimization. According to Collins and Carson, however, there is one inevitability and one possibility. Inevitably, the new relationships will be influenced by the past trauma and the ensuing survival responses. A possibility is that the family member, once a trauma victim, will become a perpetrator of trauma.[8]

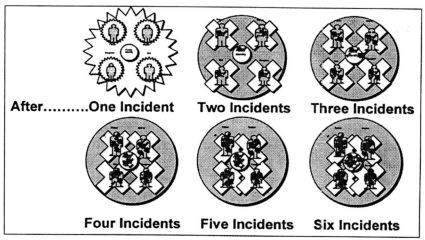

Figure 22: The Progression of Trauma in the Family.

The loss of identity caused by the trauma, along with this process of being traumatized then fighting to prevent further trauma, causes fused identity states in the family. Notice that in the progression of the trauma shown in the diagram that the family members move closer together with each incident. This represents *relationship fusion* which involves many elements, including *boundary erosion* and *projection*. According to Collins and Carson, *boundary erosion* means that:

1. Family members do not have an understanding of, or an agreement about, what constitutes appropriate interaction among themselves;

2. With the absence of such an agreement, the family members take liberties with others' lives that violate natural psychological law.

An example of something that occurs as a result of boundary erosion is "mind reading." This type of mind reading is not simply guessing what the other person thinks, nor is it some psychic process. Rather, one individual *actually believes* they *know* what the other individual(s) will think, believe, feel and respond. As mind reading continues in a relationship, both individuals become more and more isolated. In the extreme, the person doing the "mind reading" begins to have a relationship only with himself. If this "mind reader" is a perpetrator, he or she begins to take liberties with the life of the other individual—abusing, manipulating, and otherwise controlling the other's life with what he or she believes to be complete justification.

Projection is a common defense mechanism used by most people at some point in their lives. It is the process by which one individual experiences internal feelings or other concerns but perceives them as originating in someone else. For example, when you are at a theater watching a movie and you courageously approach the screen to touch Tom Cruise, you will get a hand full of nothing. He is not there, only his image. You will not even feel the film because it is behind you inside the projector. The image of Tom Cruise is projected onto the screen in front of you. Similarly, perpetrators project unwanted thoughts or feelings onto the person closest to them, perceiving them as emanating from the other individual. Perpetrators of trauma use projection in a very destructive manner.

The Chemically Dependent Perpetrator and Projection

When a chemically dependent perpetrator experiences the pain and loss caused by his or her own toxic behavior contradicting his or her values, beliefs, image and reality, he or she enters a process of projection which allows him or her to see the cause of the internal pain and loss as originating in the person closest to him or her. This person is usually a spouse but may also be a parent, child, boyfriend, girlfriend or other primary relationship. As boundary erosion continues and the perpetrator establishes the belief that he or she has the right to punish the person closest to him or her, projection accelerates the process. He or she then figuratively attacks the internal pain, which he or she now views as coming from the other person, and in the process *literally* attacks the other person verbally, physically, or sexually.

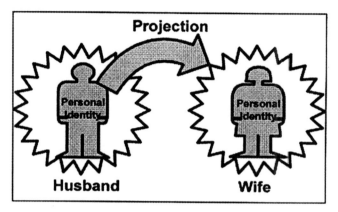

Figure 23: The Perpetrator Uses Projection

Not all chemically dependent people become violent, though statistics tell us that most violence comes from chemically dependent people. The non-violent chemically dependent person uses projection in the same manner. His or her denial of the pain and loss originating from the use of the chemical is fully supported using projection.

The Trauma Victim and Projection

Victims of trauma use projection to deal with their internally retained pain and loss also. They project internal pain onto others, thereby seeing the pain as originating in others and not in the source of the trauma—chemical dependency or sin. They also use another form of projection called *counter projection* through which they project onto the perpetrator rationales for their weird behavior. This explains the perpetrator's behavior for the victim, and results in the victim's direct support of the person who is abusing him or her.

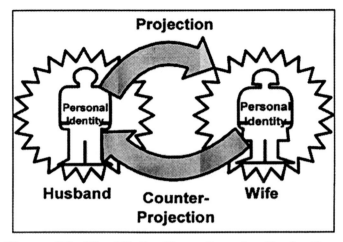

Figure 24: The Victim Uses Counter Projection.

Consider the following example. Jonathan was living with his parents while completing college. His father was an alcoholic and verbally abusive. He had been physically abusive at times in Jonathan's life, also. His alcoholic father was very controlling of 22-year-old Jonathan, requiring a 12:00 a.m. curfew, even though Jonathan worked in a restaurant that did not close until 11:00 p.m. He required Jonathan to clean the house and wash the dishes, even though Jonathan did not eat at home. One day Jonathan decided he could not take it anymore, and in the midst of an argument with his father left the house and did not return for two days. He called his father and said he was moving out to live with a friend. When Jonathan returned to get his things, he found that his father had thrown away a trunk containing his high school football trophies, letter jacket, team pictures and other high school memorabilia. His father claimed that he thought it was empty. Jonathan was crushed and furious. He left without confronting his father and blamed himself for leaving the house in such an inappropriate manner.

The alcoholic father in this illustration is projecting his internally retained pain onto Jonathan. He sees Jonathan as the source of his frustration, anger, hurt and grief. Therefore, he torments Jonathan with constant demands and unrealistic expectations. He thinks, "If only that boy would shape up, my life would be peaceful and I wouldn't drink so much." Jonathan uses counter projection to explain his father's unreasonable behavior. He thinks, "My father is stressed out because of all the jobs he's lost. It's not his fault the economy is so bad and the companies he's worked for keep downsizing. It's the government's fault. They need to do something about the economy so my father can relax. I shouldn't have left in such a hurry. I should have planned my leaving and taken everything with me the first time. He didn't know those things were important. It weighed 100 pounds. How did he lift it by himself?"

The term "codependency" has been widely used to refer to any relationship that appears unhealthy. In its original form, the term was coined to refer to individuals who were involved intimately with a chemically dependent person. They were considered to also be "dependent" on the chemical, not physically, but emotionally. Throughout this book, this narrow definition of codependency, or enabling, will be used. Specifically, codependency is the process through which a spouse or parent of a chemically dependent person projects onto the chemically dependent person a picture of how he or she used to be prior to his or her dependence. When interacting with the addict, the loved one sees the "old" person and expects them to respond in the "old" ways. The loved one is continually surprised by the addict's behavior.

Non-chemically dependent people in society use a very dangerous sort of projection. They project onto the chemically dependent people their own capacity for chemical use. In other words, drinkers who are not alcoholics expect drinkers who *are* alcoholics to be able to drink and control their consumption. This allows the non-addicted drinker to justify his or her use of alcohol or other drugs *known* to cause addiction. It also provides support for the addict to continue his or her drug use. After all, "Quitting is just a matter of willpower or choice. If I can do it, they can do it." This feeds right into a chemically dependent person's denial system. "I'll quit when I'm ready. I'm just not ready yet."

Families were created by God. He established the first couple, the first marriage, and the first family unit when he created Eve to be with Adam. From that time on, Satan has been attacking families. Since he cannot be everywhere at once to do it all himself, he sends his minions. When trauma occurs in a family, usually due to someone's sin, it plants the seeds of destruction which grow and bear fruit in that generation, and the next, and the next, and the next. Until one family unit stands up and says "No more!" it is like a boulder rolling wildly down a hillside, destroying everything in its path. If you stood in front of a rolling boulder and tried to stop it by yourself, you would be crushed. However, if God is standing with you—supporting you, living inside of you—then He, working through you, can not only stop the boulder, but can also destroy it. Are you in that family? Will *you* stand up and say *"NO MORE!"*?

Chapter Four: Survival Responses—A Different Way of Looking at Symptoms

The most significant difference between Etiotropic Trauma Management and all currently known approaches to dealing with the effects of trauma is this: Other models focus on changing or managing the symptoms. ETM focuses on the *source* of the trauma, which is contradicted existential identity. When selected symptoms are reduced, changed, or otherwise modified, other non-ETM therapists consider the treatment to have been successful. Not so with ETM. We do not consider trauma to be resolved even if symptoms have been reduced, changed, or otherwise modified. The reduction of symptoms is not a clear indicator as to whether trauma has been resolved or not. Even with diagnosable PTSD, the symptoms come and go. Sometimes they seem to be severe, other times they seem to be quite manageable or even absent. "Delayed onset" is common with PTSD. This means that days, weeks, months or even years may pass before symptoms become identifiable.

The goal of ETM/TRT is the resolution of trauma through the reconstruction of the existential identity. We believe this is accomplished through the five-phase process of TRT which precludes focusing on symptoms. For example, when you visit the doctor for a sore throat, in order to treat you properly he or she must develop his or her diagnosis. By asking questions about your symptoms and through direct observation, he or she follows a logically laid out path leading the doctor to a specific diagnosis. Many diseases, however, have similar symptoms. A sore throat can be a sign of infection, allergy or yelling too much at last night's football game. Do you have a fever? How swollen are your glands? All of these questions help to narrow the diagnosis and lead the physician to the correct treatment medications that will, hopefully, fight the infection or alleviate the symptoms. This same type of treatment is used in Psychiatry, i.e., the client describes his or her symptoms and, through descriptions and direct observation the Psychiatrist makes a diagnosis. Medication is then prescribed to, hopefully, alleviate the symptoms.

Because scientists have known so little about the brain, there has been an underlying assumption that "fixing" the problem is not possible; therefore, we will try to make the symptoms more manageable. Our knowledge about the brain is changing, however. More and more research is showing exactly what parts of the brain are affected by certain stimuli. Many researchers, including J. Douglas Bremner, now agree that trauma affects the hippocampus of the brain, which researchers believe is responsible for the sequencing of events.[9] Through his research, Jesse Collins believes that, more specifically, the synapse between the neurons in the hippocampus is the location of the trauma.[10]

What ETM is postulating is that symptoms are not only a normal response to trauma but also a necessary response in order for the person to continue on with survival. Survival is always the first order of business. Therefore, what other theorists call "symptoms," Collins and Carson have named "survival responses." You may think we are talking about reframing here, such as the difference between looking at a glass half-empty or looking at it as half-full; but it goes much deeper than that.

The paradoxical relationship that exists between the etiology of the trauma and the symptoms (survival responses) of the trauma not only keeps the victim of trauma trapped in his or her pain but also continues the *need* for symptoms (survival responses) until the etiology is reversed. When the symptoms of trauma are treated directly without recognizing the etiology of the trauma—continuous unreconciled contradicted values, beliefs, image and reality—the etiology is repressed even further. In other words, the person's thoughts that "I just need to change, this past experience has nothing to do with what is going on in my life now" is reinforced. He or she renews his or her focus on his or her performance and self-will and ignores his or her emotional pain and loss which is repressed below the surface of their conscious mind. When he or she is not able to change enough to meet his/her or others' expectations, more etiology is actually created. When the prescribed medication alleviates some of his or her symptoms, but not all of them, he or she feels hopeless and more etiology is actually created.

It is still not enough, however, just to recognize the connection between the past trauma and the current symptoms. Many therapists do that through identifying the trauma, talking about it extensively, expressing feelings about it, or using guided imagery to change the victim's perspective on it, all with the goal of changing unwanted symptoms. Since expression of feelings and changing perspectives or beliefs is not enough to reverse long-term trauma, MORE etiology is created when attempts to change symptoms are made. THIS is the paradox. The more focus placed on changing or reducing symptoms before the etiology is reversed, the more etiology is created; and therefore, new symptoms or survival responses are also developed. ETM uses TRT to keep the focus on resolution until the etiology is fully reversed.

Please understand that, while TRT keeps the *focus* on resolution, the survival responses still go away. They end when they are no longer necessary. In the ETM educational process we explain survival responses as new behaviors, new thoughts, new beliefs, and new perceptions which develop as a result of ongoing contradicted values, beliefs, image and reality. We explain that other theorists may call these same responses symptoms or defense mechanisms. While helpful at times, these survival responses may also contradict the individual's values and beliefs about what he or she should be doing, and therefore result in more loss. Clients come to understand that the underlying purposes for survival responses are to both help the person live through the traumatic event and protect the person from recognizing that the internal damage has occurred. Survival responses keep a person focused on himself or herself, or on things around him or her, and distract him or her from focusing on the inner pain and loss. As a survivor goes through the TRT process, he or she suddenly realizes that when he/she reaches the later phases, many survival responses have changed or gone away on their own without any focus or direct effort on his or her part. This is a fascinating phenomenon to witness and experience.

Collins and Carson place survival responses in four general categories. They are:

1. <u>The assumption of responsibility for traumatic events not caused by the trauma victim.</u> This occurs when the Survivor attempts to provide a sense of control within the traumatic event, when in reality the person has lost all control. This assumption of responsibility is manifested in several ways. The individual may feel guilt or shame as a response to a traumatic event caused by someone or something else. An individual may align with and even protect the perpetrator of the trauma. This frequently occurs with prisoners of war. For example, while all of the guards are holding them captive and participate in mistreating them, one may bring them extra food sometimes or smile occasionally. The POWs begin to identify with that guard and blame themselves for triggering beatings from that guard. Another manifestation is that the individual continues to stay in a trauma causing situation. For instance, abused wives frequently stay with their abusive husbands for years or leave only to return a short while later. The trauma victim may become compulsively obsessed with the perpetrator of the trauma. She spends all of her time thinking about the perpetrator, reviewing his behavior and anticipating his next move. All of these behaviors are a manifestation of the belief that the victim is somehow responsible for the behavior of the perpetrator.

   Eating disorders, such as compulsive overeating, anorexia, and bulimia, can also show up as survival responses falling into this category. When a woman or a man is sexually abused, he/she tends to think that his/her appearance, behavior, or personality attracted the perpetrator. This is another way of taking responsibility for the perpetrator's behavior. Subconsciously, he/she attempts to become unattractive. The obsession with food serves to drown the feelings and thoughts of the past abuse, and, in his/her mind, the weight gain or loss helps to prevent future abuse. As some women begin to lose weight, they report feeling panicked. They feel unsafe and out of control. They begin to overeat or starve themselves in order to regain a sense of safety. At the same time they feel guilty for overeating or under eating, and being out of control with their weight. This is quite a dilemma, as are most survival responses.

2. <u>Denial or loss of recollection that the event(s) occurred.</u> This allows the Survivor to protect the Person from the realization that

the damage to the existential and operational identity has occurred. This may be a total loss of memory of the event, like amnesia. Or, the person may forget significant details of the traumatic event. This loss of memory may last for days, months, years, or the person's lifetime. Total loss of memory for the person's lifetime is rare. Most victims do recall the trauma at some point. Frequently memories are triggered from watching a television show or movie. Sometimes when they have children, survivors recall childhood trauma. Frequently, although they have not classified what occurred to them as trauma, they recognize it as trauma when they consider the innocence of their children. More common is the rationalization and minimization of the event or circumstances leading to the occurrence of the traumatizing event. The person also may intellectualize the circumstances surrounding the event(s) to the extent that the source or sources of the trauma are ignored. This is common with alcoholism. One client recalled how angry she would get with her older brother when he would talk back to their father. Her father would then beat her brother in front of the whole family. What she realized as she wrote her incidents was that her father was drunk. While she focused on her brother's survival behavior, she minimized the source of the trauma, which was her father's toxic behavior or alcoholism. Frequently survivors focus on the non-perpetrating parent as the source of their emotional discomfort. A woman related to me how angry she was with her mother because her mother expected her to do so much around the house as she was growing up. With further questioning she disclosed that her father was an alcoholic and compulsive gambler. He abandoned them when she was 13 or 14, and mom had to work two jobs to support the family. Mom was tense and cranky and short with the children. This is what the client focused on, subconsciously minimizing the father's drunken and abusive behavior.

3. <u>Aggressive, including passive-aggressive, activity which results in the harm of others.</u> This group of survival responses is much less socially acceptable and much more harmful than many of the others. These survival responses turn the victim into a perpetrator. These survival responses help to take the focus off of the internal pain and place it on external things or people. This can include sexual and physical assault, homicide, other anti-social activities, and even suicide. Suicide is an attempt to end the pain. In

reality the person may not want his or her *life* to end but rather wants his or her *pain* to end. If that means life ends also, so be it. If life could continue on without the pain, they would most likely choose life. Aggrandizement, the acquisition of things or power to the extent that others are harmed, is another way this survival response is manifested. The individual may manipulate relationships to the extent that others are harmed. This type of survival response is difficult to pin down since the survivor, now perpetrator, is always in the background. He draws attention away from himself by getting other people to focus on each other. In the book Games People Play,[11] the author refers to this as "Let's you and she fight." Confronting a perpetrator about this kind of survival response is almost fruitless. He or she will not admit it and may not consciously be aware of his or her behavior.

I usually consider abortion as a survival response, which fits into this category. Although many people see it as trauma in itself, it does not strictly fit the definition of trauma[12] since the woman makes a *choice* to experience it. However, many people experience post-traumatic stress symptoms as a result of having an abortion once they understand what has actually taken place. In the majority of cases I have seen, prior trauma has taken place in the woman's life, and having an abortion is a response *to* that trauma in some way. For the father of the baby and for the baby, both of whom have no choice in the matter, abortion *is* a trauma and not a survival response. A lot more could be said about abortion, but that is for another text.

Not all aggressive behavior is the result of trauma. Some people become aggressive under the influence of drugs or alcohol, some because of mental illness and some because they are just mean or have prior trauma themselves. Because of their destructive nature and the potential for permanent damage to self and others, these types of survival responses must be controlled before, during and after the TRT therapeutic process, and until the internally retained trauma is resolved.

4. <u>Helping of Self and others.</u> This form of survival response has no stigma attached and may not show any outward sign that the person is actually attempting to cover internal pain and loss. Instead, most of these responses are applauded and strongly reinforced. As

survival responses, however, they accomplish the same purpose. People using this type of survival response may be considered *caretakers*. They may focus on others' problems so much they do not seem to have time to deal with their own. They may even go so far as to start organizations to try to minimize certain types of trauma causing behavior. While someone performing these types of behaviors may normally experience a lot of fulfillment and normal job frustration, an individual performing these behaviors as survival responses feels driven. He or she experiences almost a compulsive need to help, even when others do not want help. He or she may neglect other important areas of his or her life in order to help others. This is common with ministers. I have spoken with pastors who grew up in alcoholic homes. They compulsively work to help their congregations but neglect their own families and do not understand why their own families are falling apart. What makes it even more difficult is that they perceive their drive as coming from God's calling them to minister to others. How can you argue with a call from God? That makes the survival response impenetrable.

Remember that survival responses serve two *opposing* purposes, and many times they are automatic reactions to the internally retained trauma. These reactions are not necessarily conscious choices and are similar to the formation of a callous. If your foot is rubbing against your shoe every time you walk, your brain automatically directs an increase in the build up of skin cells in that area to decrease the possibility of the skin's being punctured. You do not stop and think, "Hmm, maybe I should begin to develop a callous on my left baby toe. It seems to be rubbing an awful lot." You are unaware of the callous formation until it becomes painful or unattractive. Survival responses are the same. Until they become painful or unattractive, or the survival responses just do not work anymore, they are continued with subconscious motivation.

Consciously, however, the survivor may be aware of some inconsistencies in his or her life. She may isolate herself, withdrawing from friends and family, only to develop obsessions with some relationships in which she tries to control all of the interactions or get some vague assistance. He may find himself pursuing his life goals almost obsessively, then suddenly feel trapped by inner forces trying to hold him back—what some may label as a *fear of success*. In the early stages of the trauma's repression, she may seem indifferent to her pain and loss. Later she may experience extended bouts of feelings of self-pity and self-absorption. People suffering more intense hurt may feel as though they are on a roller coaster ride, not knowing when they got on or how to get off. They try to steady themselves and live "normal" lives when, suddenly, they are plunged into depression, grief, and anger for no apparent reason.

The Survivor also develops opposing interactions with the *perpetrator*. On the one hand the person protects the perpetrator in order to avoid the recognition that the internal trauma has occurred. On the other hand the person tries to destroy the perpetrator to prevent further trauma. As I was flipping TV channels one night, I caught a perfect example of this on one of those "live" police drama shows. Two police officers drove up to a house where a domestic disturbance had been reported. A woman was screaming for help, screaming at her husband, hitting and kicking at him as the police intervened. She reported his drunken rage and displayed her bruises and cuts. The police officers began to arrest the man. They handcuffed him and headed for the car. As they reached the car, the woman's tone suddenly changed. She began to say to the police, "Don't hurt him." Then to her husband, "I'm sorry, are you okay?" Then she began to plead with the police, "Don't take him, please!" She begged and pleaded then *began attacking the police officers*, even hitting the car and screaming for her husband as they drove him away. Because of this very phenomenon, many states now have mandatory arrest for family violence rather than leaving it up to the spouse to press charges. This illustrates the paradoxical relationship which develops between the perpetrator and the survivor.

The Impact on Self-image

As the four patterns of trauma develop in an individual, their perception of themselves and others' perceptions of them are greatly altered. This happens gradually and, due to all of the repression taking place, is not readily noticeable. Since all of the loss and emotion is repressed in the identity of the individual, no one can see the damage that has taken place. What can be seen, however, are the survival responses. The survival responses will now have the greatest influence on the person's self-image and the image of him as held by others. The self-esteem of the trauma victims have already been reduced due to the trauma. As they view themselves through the overlay of the survival responses, they may even begin to think they are insane.

Most commonly, they begin to believe that they are seeing their *true selves*. They begin to believe that this is how they have always been. Focusing on this one aspect of the trauma's patterns, the survival responses, usually results in a misevaluation of the person. Survivors are labeled as obsessive, overly controlling, deceptive, liars, neurotic, narcissistic, maladaptive, codependent, irresponsible and more. Others may even begin to view the survivor as someone who is *looking* for destructive relationships, or at some deep level, thinks he or she deserves abuse, or worst of all that he or she enjoys it. This could not be further from the truth! *No one consciously chooses trauma. No one has a need to be abused.* God created all of us with a deep need to be loved, to feel significant and accepted. We spend our time looking for this love, sometimes in the wrong places. In our search for love, we come across a lot of cruel people, also trying to fill up the holes in their lives. Unlike many other forms of therapy, Trauma Resolution Therapy does not focus only on the survival responses. TRT focuses on all elements of the trauma's patterns, and in the order in which they occurred.

Multiple Sources of Trauma

When we use the term "source of trauma," we have been talking about the etiology of the trauma that is the ongoing contradicted existential identity. When applying TRT, this is used also to refer to a particular trauma-causing incident or group of incidents. There are single-incident traumas and multiple-incident traumas. A single-incident trauma occurs when a person is assaulted by a stranger just one time. A multiple-incident trauma occurs when a person is raised by an alcoholic parent. The alcoholic parent is one "source" of trauma, but many incidents occur during the time period of growing up. Some people experience trauma from many sources. For example, one TRT graduate experienced abuse as an adult from a boyfriend, and sexual abuse as a child from a male cousin. Another experienced sexual abuse as a child from a cousin, grew up with two alcoholic parents, and experienced physical, verbal and sexual abuse as an adult from a husband.

When a person has experienced multiple sources of trauma, the traumas all work together to resist any kind of assistance in resolution. Collins and Carson refer to this as an "overall survival system of diversion."[13] This is analogous to a therapeutic game where one person is placed in the center of a circle of other people holding hands. The individual attempts to break out of the circle by throwing himself at the people surrounding him. The multiple sources of trauma join together in a similar fashion, keeping the individual isolated inside and rebuffing anyone trying to get inside to help the hurting survivor.

When more than one source of trauma is experienced, each is separated from the other(s) in that the internally retained emotional pain and loss are repressed in relation to the specific incident. You may recall that as the losses occurred, chains of emotion developed. As time passed, the emotions formed streams, much like that of a string of Christmas tree lights. The phenomenon of "acceleration" and "expansion" took place.[14] However, as the streaming of emotions takes place it doesn't stop within one source of trauma; streaming takes place between the sources of trauma, also. In other words, when repression is lifted on one source of trauma, it's lifted on all. Therefore, when the individual attempts to recall one traumatic event, he or she experiences an overwhelming emotional response which, in the end, has the effect of strengthening the system of diversion.[15] At this point the person frequently withdraws from the helping experience.

Another diversionary tactic takes place when the therapeutic focus is shifted from one source of trauma to another. For example, a female client who has three sources of trauma begins focusing on the most recent source, her ex-husband's alcoholism. As the emotions and memories are triggered from this source of trauma, the emotions from other sources are triggered also. Memories of childhood sexual abuse become overwhelming and, without the structure of TRT, the therapeutic process switches to dealing with the childhood memories. The effect is twofold. One, the recent trauma is minimized and she does not complete the process of resolving the trauma induced by her ex-husband. Two, she develops and feeds the unconscious belief that, because of the childhood sexual abuse, she somehow *chose* a husband who would abuse her because that is where she felt "comfortable," or that is what she "deserved." In an unstructured therapeutic process this particular diversionary tactic runs rampant. The five-phase structured process of TRT helps to minimize this particular problem. When a client is redirected to follow the structure, most of the time he or she will make progress. Both individual and group therapy are often necessary to keep survivors of multiple sources of trauma focused on the appropriate source of trauma.

Jessica came to see me after she heard me speak at a church training seminar. She was currently involved in a relationship with a younger man

Stop Treating Symptoms and Start Resolving Trauma!

in her church and felt hopeless about her life and career. After I completed her trauma assessment, she had six sources of trauma:

1. she had been sexually abused by a family friend as a child;

2. she had been raped by a surgeon;

3. she had been raped by a date;

4. she had been raped by an acquaintance;

5. she had been sexually abused by her male psychotherapist; and

6. her ex-husband was an alcoholic and severely abusive.

Although the current relationship she was involved in consumed her, it was not abusive. Trying to change her focus from that relationship to the trauma was like trying to peel new paint off a wall. She disappeared from therapy and returned a year or so later ready to focus on the past trauma. We began writing about her ex-husband and she started into group. Again, everything else distracted her—her job, her money, her health. She was very inconsistent in her group attendance, and finally I asked her to choose to make group a priority, or quit. She chose to quit. Unlike many people with multiple sources of trauma who usually just stop coming, she came and said good-bye to her group members. About a year later she showed up in my office again. This time she was engaged to be married to a man who raped her and continued to be involved with his ex-wife. I encouraged her to leave him and write about the rape. She disappeared again. Although she was never unpleasant—we had a great rapport, and she truly believed that Trauma Resolution Therapy worked for other people—she could not keep herself focused. Later, I learned she had married the man. Eventually, she came back again and this time stayed in the TRT process. She completed that source of trauma and came back for another. While dealing with clients who have multiple sources of past trauma can be time-consuming and frustrating, educating them about TRT helps to get them through the overwhelming initial process and they can make progress even though it may be very slow.

Of the many people who have completed TRT with me, only one did not show the results that I thought should have occurred. She was referred to me by another therapist who was working in my office at the time. She remained in individual therapy with him, while in group therapy with me. The therapist had been trained in TRT and I, mistakenly, assumed he *understood* TRT. As she progressed through the phases, her behavior became more bizarre and her emotions less focused. I consulted with the individual therapist who reported that she had many other sources of trauma that were just being realized. Unfortunately, he claimed she did not yet have clear memories of these traumas. I asked him to help her stay focused on this one source until we finished. He promised he would. However, her bizarre behavior continued, even into her Phase 5 B. The things she was doing were not at all like her. After finishing, I told her that it was my belief that her individual therapy was interfering with TRT, and that if she did not have clear memories of past sexual abuse, she could not write about them. She became very angry with me. She continued with her individual therapist, who moved to another office very soon after our confrontation. Two years later she called me and asked to come in to see me. She told me that she wanted to make things right between us because she left so angry. She went on to tell me that her individual therapy *was* interfering with the TRT. She said that she believed he caused her to experience "False Memory Syndrome." She stated that she had developed many bizarre behaviors which he labeled as "body memories," and that the whole experience had almost destroyed her and her family. Although she had been in counseling with someone else following her "escape" from this therapist, she so strongly believed in TRT that she wanted to do the five-phase process on the abuse from the therapist.

When I have clients with multiple sources of trauma, I have learned that they need to continue in individual therapy as much as possible, while going through group therapy. Also, the individual and group therapist should be the same person or have a very close working relationship. If the participant is married, frequent check-ins with the spouse by the therapist are almost always necessary. Individuals with multiple sources of trauma can get through all of their sources of trauma, but it is hard work and requires a lot of attention from the therapist. People with multiple sources of trauma are, in my opinion, the main reason most doctors and therapists have given up on resolving trauma and just try to manage the most destructive symptoms. The structure of TRT, however, gives both direction and hope for those with overwhelming past trauma.

Survival Responses or Sin?

Christians respond to ETM therapists' idea of "survival responses" in several different ways. Some seem to think that by calling symptoms "survival responses," we are excusing Christians' negative behaviors, not asking them to take personal responsibility, or just allowing them to blame others for the way they act. Also, since we do not use a behavioral approach to focus on changing sinful behaviors, some believe we are being soft on sin. This is far from the truth! TRT takes the approach of facilitating change occurring from the inside-out rather than the outside-in. First, the internal trauma is resolved and, as a result, the behavior (sin) changes on its own. Jesus espoused this principle in Matthew 23: 25-28 when He said,

"You Pharisees and teachers are show-offs, and you're in for trouble! You wash the outside of your cups and dishes, while inside there is nothing but greed and selfishness. [26] You blind Pharisee! First clean the inside of a cup, and then the outside will also be clean.

[27] You Pharisees and teachers are in for trouble! You're nothing but show-offs. You're like tombs that have been whitewashed. On the outside they are beautiful, but inside they are full of bones and filth. [28] That's what you are like. Outside you look good, but inside you are evil and only pretend to be good."[16] (CEV)

What is the good of a person's looking good on the outside but having unresolved hurt, anger and even hate on the inside? Verse 26 says "...First clean the inside of a cup, and then the outside will also be clean." TRT focuses on resolving the source of the trauma first by keeping Phases One and Two structured to focus only on the source of the trauma.

Phases Three and Four change the focus to the survival responses of the survivor. This principle is expressed in James 5:16, "Confess *your* faults one to another, and pray one for another, that ye may be healed. The effectual fervent prayer of a righteous man availeth much."[17] This scripture does not say pray for one another so that you can *change*, but so that you can be healed. Sin is not being ignored, tolerated or encouraged in TRT. In fact, TRT participants identify their own sin themselves without the need of the counselor pointing it out, thereby keeping conviction between them and the Holy Spirit. And, just to make sure the person doesn't begin focusing on changing rather healing from trauma, before being allowed to read Phase 3 each individual is asked to make a commitment not to *focus* on changing until they have completed all five phases. What many people find, however, is that many of the survival responses have already changed on their own.

Denice Adcock Colson

Religious Myths about Emotional Healing

"All I need to do is just quit doing what I'm doing and be obedient to God. I shouldn't need to go to anyone else for help!" This belief keeps us stuck in our compulsive behaviors because we cannot seem to quit, but we will not go for help. We cannot see that the compulsive behaviors are just a *symptom* of the unresolved trauma and loss. God created us to be in relationship with others. Over and over again we are encouraged and even instructed to work with others to live a Christian life. God epitomizes relationship in that He is three persons as one—Father, Son and Holy Spirit.

"Why try. I can't change the way I am. God loves me anyway. I'm saved and going to heaven. Why worry about this compulsive behavior. God forgives me." This also keeps us stuck in our compulsive behavior. Yes, God does love us and will forgive us no matter what we have done, but continuing in our sin robs us of our witness, our joy, our peace, our life! Salvation is not just for heaven, it is for now. Romans 12:2 says:

> *"Do not conform any longer to the pattern of this world, but be transformed by the renewing of your mind. Then you will be able to test and approve what God's will is—his good, pleasing and perfect will."*

Trauma Resolution Therapy is a renewing of your mind. You do not have to continue to live trapped in survival responses. And yes, many survival responses are SIN.

*"**God** is going to heal me. If I do something like TRT, then I won't be showing God that I have faith in His healing ability."*

Why God seems to "deliver" some people instantaneously from the affects of past trauma, but not others, is a mystery that we will not understand until we are in Heaven. I have worked with people who, rather than use TRT, choose to continue waiting for God to instantly heal them. They seem to think that if God does not *instantly* heal them then it does not *count* as healing. They would rather continue in a miserable lifestyle than put forth any effort. We take God so for granted sometimes. We think of Him as a gumball machine—you put a quarter in, you get a gum ball out. You put the right words, faith, ritual in—you get a healing out. There is an old preacher story about a man trapped in a flood. (Stop me if you've heard it!) He climbed up on his roof and prayed for God to rescue him. Pretty soon a man in a row boat came by and said, "Jump in and I'll take you to safety." "No thanks," the man replied. "God is going to rescue me." As the water rose higher, a motorboat came along. "Jump in," the men said, "and we'll take you to high ground." "I'm okay," the man replied. "God is going to rescue me." As the water rose higher, he wondered when God was going to rescue him. He had to climb on his chimney to keep above the water. Soon a helicopter came by. Over a megaphone a man shouted, "Grab the rope and we'll pull you up!" "No thanks," the man said. "God is going to rescue me." As the water rose higher, the man drowned. When he got to heaven and stood before God, he said, "God, I trusted you and you didn't save me from drowning. Why didn't you answer my prayer? I had lots of faith in You." God replied, "I sent you a row boat, a motor boat, and a helicopter. What more did you want?!"

God heals in many ways. The way he created our bodies to heal from wounds or to fight off infection is amazing. We take that for granted. We think that it is just the way it is supposed to be; but when something goes wrong and our bodies malfunction, we think God is holding out on us. Sometimes emotional healing requires something of *us*. We have to give up something, or learn something, or make choices. Just as I would not stunt my daughter's growth by taking all obstacles out of her way as she learned to walk, then run, God does not take all obstacles out of our way as we experience emotional healing. Faith is not always waiting for God to come to us but rather moving toward God—believing that He is where He says He is, even when we cannot see Him.

Chapter Five: Completing Trauma Resolution Therapy—The Five Phase Process And How It Is Done

Before I get into the nuts and bolts of how to do TRT, allow me to make a few comments. Remember that Trauma Resolution Therapy is not a self-help program. Part of the theory is that we need someone outside of ourselves to lead us through the resolution process so that we do not become distracted. Also, this chapter in no way completely covers the technical application of TRT as written in Jesse Collins' training manual used in the Etiotropic Trauma Management Certification Workshop. It is not intended to duplicate or replace the manual but rather to summarize it. Hopefully, this will give the reader a clearer view of what ETM and TRT are all about, and he or she can make an educated decision as to whether to pursue further training or counseling. A counselor who has completed the training may want to use this chapter as a short refresher or give it to a client as part of the educational process before beginning TRT. In fact, before completing this book, I kept a file of this basic information to give as handouts to new clients. I found this very helpful and so did my clients. Now, on with the nuts and bolts.

Like all therapeutic modalities, TRT is *not for everyone*. An appropriate TRT candidate will be:

1. able to remember and identify specific trauma incidents;

2. motivated to resolve the trauma;

3. willing to complete all five phases after being educated as to what is involved in the completion process;

4. literate;

5. stable enough to follow directions and participate in the group process;

6. not taking any drugs which might interfere or drinking alcohol in any amount;

7. willing and able to make group attendance a priority as long as necessary; and

8. not suffering from an illness which requires sedating medications such as anti-psychotics, anti-anxiety and some of the older anti-depressant medications.

Once an assessment has been completed and the decision to use TRT has been made, the participant is taken through an education and orientation process. This includes basic information, such as is included in this text, as well as what types of outcomes to expect. The actual process of Trauma Resolution Therapy can take place one-on-one or in a group setting and these options are also discussed, when available. The client completes practice writings and is taught how to follow the structure, which remains the same whether TRT is completed in group or one-on-one. It is important for this process to take place with the assistance of a trained counselor who is certified in the use of Trauma Resolution Therapy.

If a person has had more than one source of trauma in his or her life, he or she must address each source of trauma fully and separately. Therefore, if a person has multiple sources of trauma, the first step is to decide which source of trauma should be resolved first. This decision should be made in collaboration with the TRT counselor. Generally, the most recent or most pressing trauma is addressed first. If a person is currently involved in a traumatizing relationship, that relationship is always addressed first. If a person is a recovering addict, the addictive behavior as trauma is most always addressed first. The participant and counselor should consult and agree on the first source of trauma to be addressed.

There are two components to each of the five phases in TRT: the written component and the reading component. Writing is in itself a great therapeutic tool. People have used writing to express emotion and clarify facts for thousands of years. Writing is the first component of all five phases of TRT. Writing usually takes place between sessions but may take place during a session. Reading always takes place with the counselor present. First let us look at the written component of Phase One, and then we will talk about the reading component.

Phase One: The Written Component

Phase One describes in writing the actual trauma-causing event or events. This is done by recalling the traumatic incidents caused by the identified perpetrator and writing each incident down on a separate sheet or sheets of paper. The incidents may be written in any order. It is not necessary to write them in chronological order. The order in which they are recalled is fine.

There are five basic rules to follow in completing Phase One writings. These are called rules rather than guidelines because it is very important that the writer follow these exactly in order to experience the resolution of the past. This is *not* journal writing, letter writing, or an "empty chair technique." This is a very specialized narrative writing and nothing else should be substituted for this step unless the therapist is working with a special population.

Here is an example of a completed Phase One incident for a person not writing about his or her own addiction:

I was in the 5th grade, about 11 years old. You picked me up from school. The car smelled like beer. I could tell you had been drinking because the radio was blaring country music, and you were slurring your words. I felt nervous. You were driving recklessly, and I felt scared. Some policemen stopped us and made you get out of the car. One made you walk around outside, and the other talked to me. I could see you stumbling and laughing real loud. Some friends rode by with their mothers. I felt embarrassed. The police put us in their car and took us to jail. They called dad to come and get me and arrested you. I felt terrified and angry at you. I felt embarrassed and confused.

A completed Phase One incident for a person writing about his or her own alcohol or drug use will appear as follows: (the differences will be discussed at the end of this section under "exceptions")

Denice Adcock Colson

We'd been married two years or more, and a group from my work invited us to a float trip in New Braunfels. Diane and I hadn't been getting along real well. We thought we'd have some fun, and it'd be like when we were dating. She asked me not to get drunk, but I told her I'd do what I wanted to do. Inside I promised myself I'd only get a good buzz. A couple of the guys I knew filled a cooler with beer, put it in its own raft, and floated it down the river. For a while Diane stayed near us, then I didn't notice her again until we were getting near the end. We were all pretty drunk and Diane was pouting and ignoring me. I started tickling her and teasing her to get her to lighten up. She just got in the car. I sat next to her in the back seat. I was still elbowing her and making comments about some of the girls in their bikinis. She looked away from me and pressed her lips together. Everyone else was quiet and looking straight ahead. I got mad, and I started shouting obscene comments out the window about some girls. Diane started asking me to be quiet. I hung out the window and grabbed at some girls at a stop light. Diane started to cry. I felt victorious. The next day I felt stupid and embarrassed. Diane refused to go to any more office parties and did not speak to me for days.

Non-chemically dependent trauma survivors should adhere to the following five rules:

Rule 1. The perpetrator of the trauma is addressed in the second-person language, "you," rather than by name or in the third person.

Example: "We were sitting in the living room and *you* became angry. *You* picked up a lamp and threw it at my head."

Using the third person language distances the writer from the emotion and reality of the incident. Using the person's name would make it seem as though we are writing a letter *to* the person. This is a narrative *about* the incident, not a letter expressing feelings *to* the perpetrator.

Rule 2. Always write in the past tense no matter how recent it feels or occurred.

By writing about the event as history you begin the process of actually putting it behind you.

Example: "We *were* sitting in the living room, and you *became* angry. You *picked* up a lamp and *threw* it at my head."

Rule 3. At the beginning of the narrative, record the approximate time and place the incident occurred. This can include the exact date and location, or the season, grade of school, approximate age, any time-defining facts that can be recalled.

Example: "***We had been married two months. We were living in an apartment in Chicago.*** We were sitting ***in the living room*** and you became angry. You picked up a lamp and threw it at my head."

Rule 4. This is an explanation of what happened. Write a factual description of the incident with as much related detail as possible. Philosophy, opinions, and rhetorical explanations should not be included.

Rule 5. Write how you felt about the incident at the time. Write your feelings simply, without couching them in terms of "you made me feel..."

Example: "I felt *scared* and *angry.*"

Putting all of the rules together, a Phase One incident writing will look like this:

It was 1982, and we had been married for two months. We lived in an apartment in Chicago. We were sitting in the living room, and you became angry. You had been drinking beer and had probably had 7 or 8. You picked up a lamp and threw it at my head. I screamed at you and ran toward the bedroom. You called me a bitch and chased me. You grabbed my arm and slapped me. I picked up a statue next to me and hit you in the head. You stumbled back and fell on the couch. After a few minutes you started laughing then got up and left the house. I felt hurt, angry and scared.

A completed Phase One incident for a person writing about his or her own alcohol or drug use will appear as follows:

I had been drinking all evening. It was the Fourth of July, 1984. Some buddies and I decided to find a car to steal. We found a red pickup and went for a joy ride. Some police spotted us because we were swerving all over the road. I was afraid we were going to crash. When they caught up with us, my friend finally stopped. There were two police cars, and the officers had their guns drawn and pointed at us. I felt terrified and thought I was going to die. They took us to jail, then called our parents. I dreaded facing my father. I was 16-years-old.

Denice Adcock Colson

For chemically dependent people writing about their own toxic behavior, Rule 1 is changed. Rather than the second person language "you," use the first person language, "I," when describing a trauma-causing event caused by your own toxic behavior. Also include a description of your chemical use, the amount and identity. The other four rules remain the same.

Exceptions

A. When writing about someone else's trauma-causing behavior, if chemical use was involved during or prior to the incident, include a description of the chemical use, if possible, and the behavioral signs of the chemical use.

Example: "You had been **smoking pot all evening**. I woke up and noticed you were gone. I found you **stumbling** around the house, talking to the furniture."

B. For Crisis Managers and Crime Victims relating incidents not involving an interpersonal relationship, you may opt for using the third person language, "he" or "she," rather than the second person language.

Example: "The car was smashed from the front and the rear. *She* was lying in the street with blood everywhere" or "*He* broke through the front door and *he* lunged at me."

After reviewing the rules, the individual is asked to write three incidents and show them to the counselor before writing any more. This is because most people do not write them correctly the first time and the counselor will need to review them and correct them. If the participant has written too many incidents and is required to rewrite them all, he or she may become discouraged and give up. However, after mastering the writing style of Phase One with the counselor's direction, the participant may write as many incidents about the identified perpetrator as he or she can remember. The participant must save all of the completed Phase One writings since they will be used in Phase Two. I recommend the use of a three ring binder. The participant must complete Phase One, writing and reading, before beginning Phase Two. Participants must not start any phase without the direction of the counselor.

Examples of Other Phase One Incidents

Stranger Assault/Robbery

It was Sept 29, 2001. It was around 8:30 P.M. and I was walking out to my car from a jewelry store. As I passed some vans a couple of guys ran out from between them and grabbed me. I felt terrified! I started screaming. One held me by the shoulders while the other grabbed my purse. The jewelry store bag was around my wrist and one of them tried to get it off. I felt like my wrist was cut or scraped and bruised, but it wouldn't come off. I had the keys in my fist in that hand and the bag handle wouldn't slide off. I kept screaming. They were cursing and threatening me. The one holding me by the shoulders said, "Shut up, bitch or I'll shoot you." The one trying to get the bag off was saying something like, "Come on, come on." People must have started running toward me because suddenly they took off with my purse but left the bag. Immediately there were people right next to me trying to help me. I heard a car squeal real loud in the parking lot. I was shaking uncontrollably. I felt terrified, confused and afraid I was going to die. I felt scared because they had my purse with my address and lots of personal information. A kind woman led me inside and we were surrounded by several other people including a security guard with a gun. I felt safer. I called my husband and he came to get me.

Home robbery

It was December 19, 2000. We came home from a Christmas party around 11:00. As we pulled into the driveway, I noticed our dog ran out of the garage when I opened the garage door. I remember thinking, "How did she get in there? Did I leave the door to the garage open?" I looked to see and it was closed. I asked my wife, "Did you let Patty into the garage?" She looked confused too and said, "No, I don't think so." Patty was a Golden Retriever and I'm sure we would have noticed had she tried to sneak past us. I felt confused and disoriented. I looked around the garage and noticed things were out of place. Could Patty have knocked down my new power tools? They seemed to be lying on the ground. I felt the hairs on my arm and the back of my neck stand up. Something inside me said, "Be careful!" My wife sat frozen in the seat next to me. I reached out and put my hand on her leg. I said a fast prayer in my head, "God help us! What should we do?!" I suddenly put the car in reverse and backed out as fast as I could. Patty followed us wagging her tail. I stopped long enough for my wife to open her door and call Patty to her. She jumped up on my wife's lap, a big Golden in the front seat of a Mercury Sable, and climbed over us to the back seat. For a few moments I felt a little hysterical and thought I would laugh or cry. Then I backed on out and headed down the street. We stopped a couple of houses down and I called the police on my cell phone. They arrived with no lights or sirens and followed us back up to our house. They walked around the house and found the back door standing open. The glass had been broken and they had reached around and opened it from the inside. I had not put the alarm on. After the police went through the house to make sure no one was there we went in to survey the damage. Everything was a mess. All of our electronics were gone. Bedroom drawers were dumped on the floor. My wife's grandmother's silver service was gone. Our computers were gone. I felt devastated. I felt guilty and responsible. I felt angry and sad. I put my arms around my wife and she cried. I felt helpless. I prayed to God to please help us and thanked Him for keeping us safe.

Verbal abuse

It was June 12, 1999. We were on our honeymoon at Disney World. We had just arrived at the hotel and were unpacking our things in our room. I felt excited to be there and a little nervous about making love later. We were chatting about how nice the room was and talking about what we wanted to do during the week. You said, "Where's my electric razor?" I said, "I don't know." You said irritably, "It was in the bag with the rest of the stuff I brought over for you to pack for me." I said, "Sorry I didn't see it". You suddenly got louder and said, "You stupid idiot, I put it in there!! What are you, blind!!??" I felt stunned and shocked. I had never heard you talk that way before. My stomach knotted and I stood frozen for a second. "Maybe it's over in that bag", I said. You stomped over to the other bag and angrily turned it upside down and dumped everything on the bed. You reached out and snatched the razor and said, "There it is. I knew I put it in my bag!" Then you went on unpacking and talking about what you wanted to do. Soon you wanted to make love. I felt numb and shocked, confused, hurt and worried. You never said anything about your outburst; you never said you were sorry. You acted as if nothing had ever happened. I felt alone, isolated and disoriented.

Car Accident

It was November 1987. I was driving home from work in my two day old, gently used (but new to me) red, Nissan 300ZX with T-tops. I was in the center lane, next to the concrete divider. There were five lanes of traffic to my right, all headed south at about 45-50 miles per hour. I noticed a lot of flashing lights ahead and off the highway on the access road. I remember thinking, "They must have had a big accident up there". I noticed a police car entering the highway, headed the same direction I was. His car seemed to pitch and swerve. I thought "He's driving too fast!" Then his car started spinning across the lanes of traffic. He spun across five lanes of traffic without getting hit and landed right in front of me facing me. I remember thinking to try to swerve to miss him, but didn't want to go into the car on the right of me or into the huge concrete dividers to the left of me. I remember thinking "I can't get around him". I felt panicked, but everything happened so fast. I felt the impact of hitting him head on. I felt my body being thrown against my seat belt hard and my head slung around. I felt like a ball in a pin-ball machine being bounced around in every direction. I heard lots of loud crashing sounds and squealing tires. When my car came to a stop I was facing north one lane to the right of the one I had been in. There were stopped cars everywhere and several seemed to be wrecked. I felt scared and very sore. My neck hurt, my back hurt, my knees hurt, my chest hurt. I had a cut on my collar bone area from the seat belt and my knees had gone through the hard plastic dash. I sat stunned while people ran up to talk to me. They pried my door open and asked if I was okay. I said, "Yes, but I hurt." They asked if I could breathe, if anything felt broken. The EMT's seemed to get there immediately. At some point I had started crying. They tried to calm me down and told me not to move. They said they wanted to get me on a back board and take me to a hospital. They asked me what had happened and I told them about the police car spinning across traffic. I asked how the policeman was and said I tried to go around him but there wasn't any room. They assured me he was fine. Everything sort of runs together from there. They strapped me on a backboard and put me in an ambulance. They drove me to a nearby hospital. I must have had them call some friends for me because they later came and picked me up. I felt discouraged, hurt, sad, angry, overwhelmed, alone, and in physical pain.

Death of a Loved One

It was a Saturday in October, 1997. I was sitting on the sofa with my husband, watching T.V. The phone rang. It was my father. He said that you had been taken to the hospital with chest pain and that he was in the emergency room waiting for you to be examined. He said he would call back when he knew something. I felt shocked and scared. I told my husband and began to cry. The phone rang again about a half-hour later. Dad said they had admitted you and taken you right to surgery. He said that the doctors were hopeful and that we should pray. He said they suspected a blockage and were doing a bypass. I asked if I should come and he said, not yet. I felt stunned and scared. I began praying and decided to pack my bags anyway. I searched for flights on the internet. Several hours later, dad called again. I could tell when I answered that the news was not good. Dad was trying to stay calm but his voice was shaking. He said that the surgery had not gone well, that there were more problems than they had anticipated. He said that you had a stroke and slipped into a coma and that the doctors said we should come. I felt numb, shaken and weak-kneed. We scheduled a flight and went to the airport. When we got to the hospital, Dad was crying. We went in to see you. You looked pale, weak and disheveled. You looked so small. I felt helpless, sad, broken-hearted and scared. I sat by your bed all night. After several days, the doctors said that you had no brain activity. After talking to Dad, we decided to take you off of life support. You passed way only minutes after the tubes were removed. I felt sad, angry, broken-hearted, and mad at God, regretful, helpless and depressed. You were only 55 years old.

The Reading Process

The second component of all five TRT phases is the reading process. Many clients come in after completing their writings for the first time and say, "Well I wrote it, but it didn't really do anything for me." That is fine! Writing is really only required to get the facts and feelings on paper so that you can read them without introducing survival responses of analysis and avoidance. Writing the incident is not enough to resolve trauma. It must be read out loud with the TRT structure in place in order to receive the full benefit. Other people come in having had very emotional experiences while writing. Either response is normal and to be expected, but the reading is still vital.

Before being allowed to read a correctly written incident, it is very important that the participant understand the structure of the reading process. This structure remains the same whether the reading is done one-on-one with a counselor or in a group-counseling setting. In an individual session all the time may not be devoted to the TRT reading process. The session may start out with, "How have things been this week?" or other more traditional, though not client centered, counseling questions. Client centered questions like "What would you like to focus on today?" turn control of the session over to the client and undermine the structure of the

TRT process and do not belong in any part of a TRT individual or group session. Usually toward the beginning of the session I will ask, "Did you get some writing done this week? Can I see it?" Or for more advanced clients, "Do you have something to read this week? How many?" Then the rigid structure begins. It goes like this:

1. (counselor) What are you feeling about reading?

2. (participant) Nervous, anxious, but ready.

3. (counselor) Please read slowly. Read just what is written, don't add anything or stop to make comments or explanations. When you are done, lay your paper in your lap and sit quietly and don't say anything until I ask you to. You may begin when you are ready.

4. (participant) Reads incident. If the person reads too fast, counselor interrupts and slows them down as many times as needed. Specialized techniques are taught in the Certification workshop. It is not unusual for the person to cry and need time to pull himself or herself together.

5. (counselor) When the participant finishes, the counselor uses discretion as to when to say, "What are you feeling?"

6. (participant) "Hurt, sad, really angry and stupid."

7. (counselor) "As you were reading, I felt" .... The counselor inserts empathetic feelings focused on the perpetrator, for example, "I felt betrayed, used, hurt and insulted."

8. (participant) The participant is instructed in advance to respond with "thank you." No discussion or questions are allowed here.

9. (counselor) "What are you feeling?"

10. (participant) "I feel betrayed and used and still angry."

11. (counselor) At this point the counselor may let the participant read another incident and repeat steps 4-10 or move on to "observational feedback." Moving on to observational feedback would signal the end of the reading process. Observational feedback means that the counselor gives physical observations of the participant without

any emotional interpretation. For example: "I noticed that your eyes turned red and you cried. I noticed your hands shook and your feet were tapping." The counselor would never say, "I noticed you were sad or angry," as that would be interpreting the client's feelings for him or her. While this is a part of traditional client-centered therapy, it is not a part of the TRT reading process.

12. (participant) Again the participant is instructed in advance to respond with "thank you. No discussion or questions are allowed here, either.

13. (counselor) "What are you feeling?"

14. (participant) "Still angry, but relieved, tired, and sad."

15. (counselor) "Thank you for reading, Sara." Let's take a deep breath.

16. (participant) Takes a deep breath and the reading process is finished.

This structure is very important and is designed to keep the client in his or her feelings and not in his or her head. Analyzing the incident does not move the resolution process along at this point. Identifying it and grieving over it does. Again, this is a simplified version since all types of variables happen when actually going through the process. However, deviation from the structure is not allowed in the TRT process.

The same process takes place in group but on a grander scale. Since there are more participants who must interact with each other during a ninety-minute group, all the time is structured to avoid mishaps.

There are four basic stages in the TRT group process. First the facilitator asks each group member to "Check-in." During this time each group member briefly states how he or she is feeling at that moment. Common responses are "rushed," "nervous," "tired," etc. Also, since many participants are seen only in group, if any extraordinary events have occurred that the counselor needs to know about, i.e., the death of a loved one, etc., they are disclosed during this time so that individual sessions can be scheduled.

Next the facilitator leads the group through processing the previous week's session. Each person who read the previous week is led through the process. The facilitator will ask, "Kim, briefly summarize what you read about last week," then "What did you feel after the reading? Did anything related to it come up for you that evening or during the week?" After she finishes responding, each group member is asked to share with the reader his or her feelings after the reading, any ways he or she could relate to what was read, or any memories triggered by the reading. Since no discussion is allowed during the actual reading process, this is when a group member can say, "Something just like that happened to me, and when you read that last week I felt like I was going to explode!" This part of the process provides for continuity from week to week and allows the clients to identify with each other more specifically. Also, not all of the grieving takes place in the group. This allows the facilitator as well as the group members to hear about the participants' grieving experiences outside of group and helps the participants to tie the grieving experiences to the reading process. Try to keep this part brief, however.

After everyone has had an opportunity to share, the facilitator will ask, "Who wants to read tonight?" If more than one person came prepared to read, I will ask, "Who's going first?" In a working group of six to eight members, it is not unusual to run out of time. I have even had people draw numbers and set up a queue for the next week. Working groups are anxious to read and get through the process. New groups, however, take time to get moving. We will frequently end early for the first few months.

After a reader is chosen, the facilitator will ask everyone else to place anything he or she is holding on the floor and to give complete attention to the reader. The focus should remain on the reader for the duration of his or her reading and processing. The facilitator asks, "Kim, what are you feeling about reading tonight?" The reader will give a brief answer, usually something like nervous, or embarrassed, or calm. The facilitator then instructs the reader, "Read slowly, speak up so everyone can hear. You can start when you are ready, and turn the paper over or close the book to let us know when you are finished." The reader then proceeds to read the incident from beginning to end, just as it was written, with no comments or explanations. Many times people feel the need to stop and cry or hesitate. Usually the group sits quietly, grieving with the person. Offering tissue or touching can be disruptive to the flow of emotion and is discouraged. I place a box of tissue in the center of the circle where it can be reached by everyone.

When the reader has finished, the facilitator will ask, "What are you feeling, Kim?" The reader responds with feeling words like angry, hurt, sad, disappointed, etc. It is the facilitator's job to help the person stay focused on the perpetrator rather than on herself. Words like "ashamed" or "guilty" usually mean the reader is focusing on her response to the trauma. Reminding the reader to focus on the perpetrator by saying, "What do you feel about your mother's behavior, Kim?" usually helps shift the focus.

After the reader has said as much as she wants to, the facilitator asks the rest of the group, "What did you feel about what Kim read?" Notice the use of "what" rather than "how." This gets the group members to use more feeling words and to stay focused on the reader rather than on themselves. Each group member will look the reader in the eye and express his or her feelings. No giving of advice, judgment or blaming of the reader is allowed.

When the group member is finished, the reader responds simply with "thank you." A verbal acknowledgment is important to help prevent shock and withdrawal in the reader. After all group members have finished, the facilitator returns to the reader to ask, "What are you feeling?" Sometimes the reader may identify with the feelings expressed by the rest of the group, or she may feel the same as before.

When the reader has finished expressing her feelings, the process is repeated if she has another reading. If not, the facilitator moves on to observational feedback by asking the group, "What did you observe while Kim was reading?" Group members take turns making physical observations, without interpretation. In other words, they express only what they saw, not what they think the person felt. Examples include, "I noticed you were clinching your hands into fists," "I noticed you cried," "You laughed when you read the first line," etc. It is very important for the facilitator to help the group members stick with observations only and allow the reader to interpret the behavior for herself. This gives the reader practice in identifying her feelings and prevents a conflict between members. It also affirms to the reader that people were paying attention to her. When observations have been made, the facilitator again returns to the reader to ask, "What are you feeling?"

Then the facilitator thanks the reader for sharing her story with the group. The facilitator asks everyone to take a deep breath, stretch and then goes on to the next reader. After all readings for the night are complete, the group stands for a group hug and/or prayer and dismisses until the next week.

Stop Treating Symptoms and Start Resolving Trauma!

This process is followed regardless of the phase. The only exception is Phase Five B, the graduation and celebration phase.

We have been looking at the TRT group process as if through a pair of binoculars in order to see even the minutest detail. Now let us turn the binoculars around and get a wider view of a TRT group. Here you have a group of individuals all going through the TRT five-phase process, all writing uniformly about either their own addictions or the perpetration of someone else on their lives. They may enter the group at different times and each person works at his or her own pace. Therefore, each may be in a different phase. There may be a few in Phase One, a couple in Phase Two, one in Phase Three, one in Phase Four and one ready to do Phase Five B. The group is closed in that no visitors are allowed and a person must come through the facilitator to participate. The group is open-ended in that there is no time limit; people come and go as they start and finish the five-phase process. I have had group participants take anywhere from six months to two years to complete all five phases, depending upon how many incidents they had to write about, how intense the trauma was, and how faithfully they attended and did their homework. However, the *structure* is consistent. The *structure* remains the same. The *structure* is what the participants depend on each week as they return to resolve their sources of trauma.

Phase Two

Phase Two begins the objective analysis of each incident. Up until this point the person has focused on his or her feelings about the traumatic events. Now the incident is broken down to include contradicted values, beliefs, image and reality; the person's losses, and his or her thoughts and behaviors in response to the incident (survival responses). The first step is to arrange all of the Phase One incidents in chronological order. Then the following form or "matrix" is completed for each incident.

SUMMARY OF TRAUMA CAUSING EVENT	SUMMARY OF FEELINGS	VALUES, BELIEFS, IMAGE AND/OR REALITY CONTRADICTED BY THE INCIDENT	LOSSES EXPERIENCED BECAUSE OF THE CONTRADICTIONS	THOUGHTS, BEHAVIORS IN RESPONSE TO THE INCIDENT (SURVIVAL RESPONSES)

Column 1 is a brief summary of the traumatic incident. For example, this may be: "I was 15 years old. You were drunk and sexually abused me in the living room while Mom was at work." The summary should be kept brief but distinctive. "Incident #1" is not enough. Rewriting the entire incident is too much.

Column 2 is a simple copying exercise. Copy all of the feelings listed in the Phase One incident into this column. There is no need to duplicate feelings. If you think of other feelings, you may list them now.

Column 3 takes some thought and concentration. Ask yourself, "What *should* my perpetrator have been doing?" or "How *should* I have been treated?" In this column you put into words what made the act of the perpetrator wrong in your mind. The focus stays on the perpetrator, not on the victim. For example, you may write: "Fathers should not touch their daughters sexually" or "I should have been allowed to grow up and make a choice about my first sexual activity." Something like "I should have trusted my father" does not belong here since it switches the focus to the victim. This statement can be rephrased as "My father should have been trustworthy." Write as many values and beliefs contradicted by this incident as you can recall. Do not just write a few to have something in the column. The more thorough you are, the more effective the treatment.

Column 4 lists all of the losses related to the previous contradictions. For example, since the father's behavior contradicted the belief that fathers should be trustworthy; one loss would be "trust." You would also list things like innocence, good judgment, the opportunity to be a virgin on my wedding night, faith in God, etc. Again, any and all losses you can think of should be listed.

Column 5 gives you the opportunity to finally list what you thought and did in response to the trauma. In this column the focus begins to shift to the victim, although the emphasis is on the incident triggering these responses. This is what the victim did to survive. List those thoughts and behaviors directly related to the specific incident. General responses will be listed later. Examples would be: "I began to avoid my father," "I lied about the bruises," "I lied to get out of the house," etc.

The completed form will look something like this:

SUMMARY OF TRAUMA CAUSING EVENT	SUMMARY OF FEELINGS	VALUES, BELIEFS, IMAGE AND/ OR REALITY CONTRA- DICTED BY THE INCIDENT	LOSSES EXPER- IENCED BECAUSE OF THE CONTRA- DICTIONS	THOUGHTS, BEHAVIORS IN RESPONSE TO THE INCIDENT (SURVIVAL RESPONSES)
I was 15 yrs old. You were drunk and sexually abused me in the living room.	sad, scared, hurt, ashamed, angry, disgusted	Fathers should not touch their children in sexual ways	Innocence, trust, opportunity to be a virgin on my wedding night, good judgment, self-esteem	Avoid my father, avoid my friends, think you were sick, think I was a slut, became promiscuous with boys.
		I should have been allowed to grow up and make a choice about my first sexual activity.	Faith in God, trust in men, security, femininity, sexuality, respect for you, respect for myself,	Lied about the bruises, lied to get out of the house, thought it was my fault, thought it was my mom's fault
		My father should have been trustworthy.	Joy, happiness, faith in my father, my father, trust in my mother	hid your alcohol, stayed in my room unless mom was home
		Fathers should not get drunk.		

For a person writing about his or her own alcohol or drug addicted behavior, the incident might look like this:

SUMMARY OF TRAUMA CAUSING EVENT	SUMMARY OF FEELINGS	VALUES, BELIEFS, IMAGE AND/OR REALITY CONTRADICTED BY THE INCIDENT	LOSSES EXPERIENCED BECAUSE OF THE CONTRADICTIONS	THOUGHTS, BEHAVIORS IN RESPONSE TO THE INCIDENT (SURVIVAL RESPONSES)
I was driving home from work drunk and I got my 2nd DUI.	Scared, humiliated, angry, ashamed, hurt	I shouldn't have been drinking and driving again.	Self-esteem, safety, respect for myself,	drink more and secretly, smoke marijuana,
		I should learn from my mistakes.	Respect for police, my family's respect for me,	call into work sick a lot, ignore my wife, lie,
		Alcohol is not the way to deal with stress.	My car, my driver's license, my freedom, relationship with my wife, relationship with God.	Avoid my children, refuse to attend church, avoid my friends, go out with other drunks
		I would not want my daughter driving on the highway with a drunk.		,
		I should not fight with police.		

Just like in Phase One, after the facilitator has taught the participant how to complete the matrix, the participant should complete only three and then bring them in and have the facilitator look over them before writing more or reading any. I am constantly reminded of a former group member who never let the group forget that she had to re-read 20 incorrectly written Phase Two incidents after another TRT facilitator missed looking over them. I caught them when I first took over the group. She was acutely aware of the difference when she read them correctly, however.

Phase Two incidents are read in chronological order three to seven or eight at a time. The amount is left up to the discretion of the TRT counselor and the desire of the TRT participant. They should be read in a way that is not too overwhelming and allows the individual to process each incident while seeing the big picture. It also shows clearly the link between the trauma incident and the change in the individual's behavior and thought processes. The group format remains the same regardless of the phase of each individual. More specific instructions, as well as role-play opportunities, are given in the Etiotropic Trauma Management Certification Workshop.

Phase Three

In this Phase the focus has shifted completely from the perpetrator to the victim. The first maze of emotional circuitry and loss has been disassembled, and now we are addressing the second maze which was created by the individual's own survival responses. This is a simple copying exercise. Copy all of the Phase Two, column fives onto sheets of notebook paper, leaving the left margin blank for use in Phase Four. As you copy, any thoughts or behaviors that had been combined into one sentence should be separated. For example: "I hated and resented you" would be separated into "I hated you" and "I resented you."

PHASE TWO: Changes to →	PHASE THREE:
THOUGHTS, BEHAVIORS IN RESPONSE TO THE INCIDENT (SURVIVAL RESPONSES)	I avoided my father.
	I avoided my friends.
Avoid my father, avoid my friends, think you were sick, think I was a slut, and became promiscuous with boys.	I thought you were sick.
	I thought I was a slut.
	I became promiscuous with boys.
Lied about the bruises, lied to get out of the house, thought it was my fault, thought it was my mom's fault	I lied about the bruises you gave me.
	I lied to get out of the house.
	I thought it was my fault.
	I thought it was my mom's fault.
hid your alcohol, stayed in my room unless mom was home	I hid your alcohol.
	I stayed in my room unless mom was home.

After copying all the survival responses listed in Phase Two, column 5, list any other survival responses which you may not have been able to connect to a specific incident but which you suspect began as a result of the trauma. Example:

    Generally:

- I began to binge eat.

- I drank heavily in college.

- I avoided having sex with my husband.

After completing the Phase Three list, the participant reads it in one sitting, straight through without any interruptions. The group structure remains the same with feelings processed following the reading. Before the participant reads, it is very important that the facilitator request the participant to make an agreement that he or she will not use this list to focus on trying

Stop Treating Symptoms and Start Resolving Trauma!

to change his or her behaviors until he or she has finished all five phases. This helps to keep the participant focused on the resolution process and not on changing his or her survival responses. Most participants find that many of the survival responses they read about have already changed on their own, to some extent.

Phase Four

In Phase Four the participants will be summarizing their survival responses and placing them in a matrix similar to Phase Two's matrix. The first step is to summarize or group the survival responses listed in Phase Three. One way of doing this is—using the Phase Three document—begin at the top, and assign a number to each new behavior on the list. Give similar behaviors the same number until all behaviors have been assigned a number.

PHASE THREE:

1. I began to avoid my father.
1. I began to avoid my friends.
2. I began to think you were sick.
3. I thought I was a slut.
4. I became promiscuous with boys.
5. I lied about the bruises you gave me.
5. I lied to get out of the house.
3. I thought it was my fault.
6. I though it was my mom's fault.
7. I hid your alcohol.
1. I stayed in my room unless mom was home.

Generally:

8. I began to binge eat.

9. I drank heavily in college.

1. I avoided having sex with my husband.

10. I criticized my children for asking any questions about sex.

After assigning numbers to all of the survival responses, group together those with the same number and write a summary statement for each group.

1. I withdrew and avoided contact with everyone in my life.

2. I thought insulting thoughts about my father.

3. I thought insulting thoughts about myself.

4. I became sexually promiscuous.

5. I lied to everyone to cover up.

6. I blamed my mother.

7. I began to try to control my father.

8. I used food as a comfort.

9. I drank to avoid my feelings and memories of the abuse.

10. I blamed my children for making the memories return.

Next, list the summary statements in column one of the Phase Four matrix and complete columns 2 and 3. This is very similar to Phase Two, except that the focus is now on the victim/survivor. It is important for the participants to list as many things as they can think of in columns 2 and 3 rather than just putting something in the column. The more thorough the participants are, the more effective the treatment will be.

SUMMARY OF SURVIVAL RESPONSES	VALUES, BELIEFS, IMAGE, AND/ OR REALITY CONTRADICTED BY THE RESPONSE	LOSSES RESULTING FROM THE CONTRADICTIONS
I withdrew and avoided contact with everyone in my life.	I should interact with others in an open and honest way.	Friends, intimacy, security, self-esteem, love, opportunities to have fun,
	I should have intimate relationships.	Sense of belonging,
	I should not hide things from my friends.	
I thought insulting thoughts about my father.	I should love my father, I should show respect for him, I should honor him in my mind.	Relationship with father, self-esteem, respect for father, blessings from God, relationship with God,

Phase Five A

This is the summarizing phase. For Phase Five A the participants will list all of their losses from column four of Phase Two and column three of Phase Four. They will categorize the losses as either individual losses, relationship losses, or systemic (family) losses. Individual losses are personal or internal such as self-esteem, self-respect, confidence, joy, innocence, etc. Relationship losses are external or between two persons such as trust, respect, relationship with God, trust in mother, etc. Systemic or family losses are losses that a system, such as a family, experienced in common. For example: family pride, fun times, future vacations together, etc.

Column four of Phase Two will be listed on the following form:

As a result of the trauma, I experienced the following losses:

Individual losses of:	Relationship losses of:	Family Losses of:
innocence	trust	family pride
opportunity to be a virgin on wedding night	faith in God	fun times
good judgment	respect for dad	respect for dad
security	trust in men	
self-esteem	faith in father	
femininity	father	
sexuality	trust in mother	
joy	respect for self	
happiness		

Column three of Phase Four will be listed on the following form:

As a result of my attempts to survive, I experienced the following losses:

Individual losses of:	Relationship losses of:	Family Losses of:
security	friends	time together
self-esteem	intimacy	future as a family
sense of belonging	love	
	opportunities for fun	
	relationship with father	
	respect for father	
	blessings from God	
	relationship with God	

After completing the forms, participants read them in one sitting in group. Emotional reactions to 5A are mixed. Some people continue to feel very sad, while others do not have many strong feelings. Either is normal since the second maze of emotional circuitry and loss is disassembled for most people after completing Phase Four.

Phase Five B

Phase Five B is a celebration! In this phase the participants are asked to look at who they are as persons, who God created them to be, and who they *are now* as compared to what they *had to do* in order to survive. The trauma came into their lives, and they got off of the path God had laid out for them. Now they are back on the right track, or, if they have more traumas to resolve, closer to the right track. Each person in the group prepares something for the individual which represents how he or she views them. The individual also prepares something that represents how he or she views himself or herself now as compared to before he or she resolved the trauma. Many of the group members may have been together since the beginning of their trauma work, so they have probably come to know each other quite well. The changes they have seen can be reflected in their presentations. People are encouraged to be creative in this phase. Group members can write a letter, a poem, a song, sing a song, play a tape, buy a gift, paint, draw, perform a skit, make a video tape, do a demonstration, involve the whole group, or bring in whatever creative article they wish, to convey their view of the individual or themselves. The group members come prepared to send whatever they have constructed home with the graduate.

In the past one group member demonstrated how to make recycled paper, and then put a piece of it in a picture with a poem to represent the changes in herself. One group member made a video of herself performing a dance. Others have performed skits, played songs, written letters, sang, or purchased small gifts that are representative of their feelings and beliefs.

I encourage members to think and pray about what they are going to do before completing their project. Inevitably, there are one or two themes which pervade the entire Phase Five B experience, even though the group members do not get together and discuss what they will do beforehand. This phase involves a lot of *happy* tears, hugs and congratulations.

Phase Five B is scheduled two to three weeks in advance in order to give everyone plenty of time to prepare. Also, the therapist must select a day in which everyone will be present. If someone becomes ill, the 5B is postponed unless it is absolutely impossible to postpone. On the night of the 5B, no other trauma work is done in that group. All of the focus remains on the graduate. The group process is also rearranged. The group begins as usual with check-in, then processing the previous week's group. Then you move directly into the celebration. After giving instructions, the facilitator moves a chair into the center of the circle and the "graduate" is seated in the chair. Each group member then volunteers when he or she is ready to present his or her gift. The graduate moves his or her chair to sit directly facing the individual making the presentation. After the presentation, the two may shake hands, or hug or the graduate may just say, "Thank you." This process is relatively unstructured. After all group members have made their presentations, the graduate returns to his or her seat and makes his or her presentation. Usually the group leader does not prepare anything but does say a few words on behalf of the graduate's progress in group. The group is then ended with a group hug, as usual.

One word summarizes the TRT process—structure. Without the structure, it is not TRT. If someone is using a different structure, i.e., adding another phase, writing the five most difficult incidents of trauma in Phase One rather than all of them, using confrontation in the group process, etc., then it is not TRT. A trained TRT counselor learns the structure, trusts the structure, and follows it to the letter so that a TRT participant can learn the structure, trust the structure and follow it to the letter. When there are no outside interferences, the structure works.

Chapter Six: What Does TRT Accomplish?

People enter Trauma Resolution Therapy in various ways. Some come alone; some come with family members in tow. Some of the variations include:

1. An individual entering TRT to resolve trauma which is no longer occurring and they have little or no contact with the perpetrator. Example: Sue entered TRT to write about her alcoholic father who had passed away five years ago. Mary wrote about a rape from a stranger that occurred when she was fourteen years old.

2. An individual entering TRT to resolve past trauma and he or she continues to live with or have regular, close contact with the perpetrator. Example: Tanya entered TRT to write about her ex-husband who was a cocaine addict. Although he was sober and no longer abused her, she continued to talk to him and see him because of their children.

3. An individual entering TRT to resolve trauma which is ongoing and he or she continues to live with or have regular, close contact with the perpetrator. Example: Angela entered TRT to write about her current alcoholic boyfriend with whom she continued to live. He continued to drink and perpetrate her.

4. A couple entering TRT, both working on past trauma, neither are perpetrators. Example: Joe and Leslie entered TRT to both write about past childhood trauma.

5. A couple entering TRT, one working on past trauma of having perpetrated the other partner in the past, the other working on the partner's perpetration. Example: Jennifer and Mike entered TRT together. He wrote about his past alcoholic behavior and she wrote about his past alcoholic behavior.

6. A couple entering TRT, one working on past trauma, the other having no history of trauma in his or her life, but attending couples' sessions for support. Example: Renee entered TRT to write about her ex-husband's abusive behavior and her current husband Jim attended couples' sessions to become educated on the TRT process and support Renee.

7. A couple entering TRT, both working on ongoing trauma, both perpetrating each other. Example: Terri and Mike entered TRT, both alcoholics but now sober, but continuing in verbally and physically abusive behavior toward each other.

8. A couple entering TRT, both working on ongoing trauma, neither are perpetrators. Example: Jim and Nancy entered TRT to write about their drug-addicted son who had also been diagnosed with bipolar disorder.

Other variations include families entering TRT to write about a mutual near-death experience, or the death of a family member, or the birth of a handicapped child. More and more we are seeing couples with one or both spouses experiencing on-the-job trauma related to terrorism fears. Trauma comes in all shapes and forms.

The TRT Five-Phase process for long-term trauma is the same regardless of the scenario surrounding the person's life. However, if a person enters TRT who is still in a relationship with the perpetrator, completing the five phases is *much* more difficult. Many perpetrators interfere with the survivor's attempts to get help. One woman was writing about her husband who was an active crack addict. He would take the car, promising to bring it back in time for her to go to group, then not show up until an hour later. Also, the continuation of the perpetration means the person continually has new incidents about which to write. Stephanie had completed all of the incidents she could remember from the past, but her husband kept doing new things. She became very frustrated with the process. In order to get her into Phase Two, we combined individual and group sessions, having her write or tell the recent incidents in Phase One style during an individual session and then put them into the Phase Two matrix which she continued to read in group.

As a survivor goes through the TRT process, he or she will set boundaries for the perpetrator, refuse to allow the projection to continue, and the perpetrator will begin to have to deal with his or her own feelings and behavior. It is possible that at this time the perpetrator will ask for some help and enter treatment. It is also possible that the perpetrator will switch their projection to someone else, such as a parent or someone with whom he or she is having an affair. If the latter occurs the perpetrator's chances of getting help are very slim. It is also possible that the survivor will decide he or she has had enough and leave both the trauma and the perpetrator.

Separation frequently occurs when the perpetrator does not change and the survivor resolves the past trauma. For Christians, this can be another double-bind situation. On the one hand, living with an abuser contradicts his or her values and beliefs about what he or she should be doing, but on the other hand, divorce also contradicts his or her beliefs about what he or she should be doing. Many pastors and religious leaders, even today, will not recommend separation to a woman who is being abused by her husband. Many more pastors recommend it now, however, than did ten years ago.

Survival responses which take on a religious tone are very common when a woman is considering divorcing an abusive husband. One woman I worked with believed God was telling her to stay with her alcoholic husband even though he had rented a separate apartment, had a girlfriend, and sat in a session with her saying, "I want a divorce. I am not coming back." He fed the illusion, however, by continuing to sleep at the house when it was convenient for him and just dropping by to see the kids whenever he chose. Trying to convince her that it was time to let go would have been an exercise in futility.

In TRT, talking someone into giving up his or her survival responses *is not done*. Instead, the therapist encourages the patient to do the writing in Phase One, which will process them out of their shock and denial stages of grief. Unfortunately, some people refuse to do the writing "because God told them they shouldn't dwell on the past." Believe me, you cannot argue with God! This is the trump card and when it is played, you might as well give up.

What to Expect

Remember that there are four patterns in the development of trauma in an individual:

Initial Effects

Pattern 1: Your experience of the initial event contradicts your values, beliefs, image and reality.

Pattern 2: The contradictions resulting from your experience of the initial event result in loss. Losses include tangibles and intangibles such as self-esteem, self-respect, respect for the other person, innocence, sense of safety, femininity, masculinity, childhood, etc. These losses—along with the emotions accompanying them—are then repressed.

Life-Long Effects

Pattern 3: The repressed losses that originate from the initial trauma foster the development of survival responses. These are new thoughts, behaviors and perceptions that, although helpful at the time, may also contradict your values, beliefs, image and reality.

Pattern 4: Survival responses that contradict your values, beliefs, image and reality create more loss. These additional losses—along with the emotions accompanying *them*—are also repressed.

Patterns one and two, the Initial Effects, are addressed in TRT Phases One and Two. Patterns three and four, the Life-Long Effects, are addressed in TRT Phases Three and Four. Phase Five is a summarizing phase which finishes the job of pointing the person toward the future and putting the trauma in the past.

Remember that the Survivor is in a dilemma. The survival responses serve two opposing purposes. One is to keep the trauma repressed, and two is to keep the trauma from occurring again.

Stop Treating Symptoms and Start Resolving Trauma!

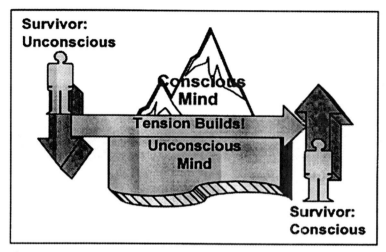

Figure 25: The Constant Tug-of-war.

The underlying need for the survival responses, however, is to protect the person. Therefore, TRT circumvents this dilemma by using the structure of the TRT process, as well as the TRT group process, to provide protection for the person. This allows the Survivor to relax and give up the need to assume the responsibility for protecting the person.

When a person enters Phase One of TRT, by writing his or her incidents as outlined, he or she identifies the specific perpetrator and specific trauma events which have occurred in his or her life. As he or she reads these incidents, he or she experiences and expresses emotions attached to the losses which occurred. He or she also begins moving through the cycle of grief. Sadness, embarrassment, and anger are emotions commonly expressed as a person writes and reads his or her Phase One incidents. Many people enter Phase One thinking that it will be an exercise in recall and that they will not be very emotional. They are truly surprised when they actually start crying! As they process out of the Shock stage of grief, they begin to experience many emotions that they have been avoiding for years. They become sad; they cry a lot—even the men. They cry at television shows, movies, even commercials. Michael came to group and asked why he was getting more depressed. As we discussed what was going on, I pointed out that clinical depression was defined by constricted emotion or lack of emotion. He was feeling a wide variety of emotion, and that which he was calling *depression* was actually *sadness*. He had long ago lost the ability to identify sadness. *It is normal to feel sad!* Anyone who had experienced the type of losses that he had experienced would feel extremely sad.

Moving through TRT Phases One and Two, a person experiences what Collins and Carson call the "Grief Cliff."[18] As you begin the resolution process, it is like you are pushing a huge boulder up a hill. At first it does not seem too difficult, but it gets harder as the incline gets steeper. You begin to get tired and want to give up. Then suddenly, the bottom falls out. People say to me, "I don't know when it happened, but suddenly I feel lighter, less burdened." They have "pushed their boulder over the cliff." There is a saying which goes "with all growth comes resistance." This also applies to resolving trauma. The emotions that have been repressed for years are now bubbling up to the surface and bursting on the scene. This is uncomfortable for trauma survivors who have been keeping the same emotions repressed for years. I remind my group members that, if you are feeling bad, then you are making progress. Because you started out in the shock stage of grief, you were, for the most part, numb to the trauma. Now you are headed for the anger stages. *Of course you are going to feel bad*! If you keep going, however, you *will* get to resolution. Emotions cannot kill you. You *are* stronger than your emotions.

As a person completes TRT Phase Two, he or she is keenly aware of the specific losses he or she experienced during the trauma. He or she begins to get extremely angry. Initially, the person becomes more irritable. Then, he or she gets *angry*, and then finally, *furious*. Although anger outbursts are common prior to starting the resolution process, this anger is different. It begins to get more focused on the perpetrator and on anyone violating his or her boundaries. People begin to set boundaries with others without being told by others what limits are needed. Initially the person may go a little overboard, like the television portrayal of a woman just returning from an assertiveness training seminar. They may return things to stores and chew out clerks, or confront waiters or family members. This will settle down, however, and the person will become more balanced in his or her approach to setting boundaries. I always warn the husbands of TRT women to expect some additional anger and sensitivity from their wives during this time. I also assure them that, if she continues in the group, it will pass.

After completing Phase Two, a person usually feels a certain amount of relief, not only because Phase Two is over but also internally, the first maze of emotional circuitry and loss has been disassembled.

Stop Treating Symptoms and Start Resolving Trauma!

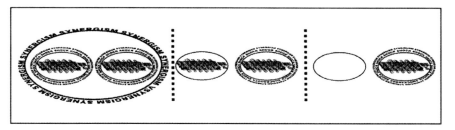

Figure 26: The First Maze is Disassembled.

Phase Three shifts the focus from the perpetrator to the survival responses of the trauma victim. Sadness, grief, and regret all become more prominent emotions. While the individuals feel guilty over some of their survival responses, shame is no longer hindering their progress. They no longer feel any responsibility for the trauma itself. They are very clear as to what happened to them and who, or what, was the cause of all of their losses. However, facing the aftermath is also very painful. The person is now moving from the anger stages of the grief cycle into the acceptance-of-the-pain stage. Crying, mourning, and deep grieving characterize this stage. The person is experiencing the pain that resulted from his or her attempts to survive.

Phase Four intensifies the pain and is, in my experience, the most difficult phase to complete. Not only is it more complicated to write but also facing the feelings associated with the consequences of survival responses is emotionally intense. Many people cry more when reading this phase than they did in any other phase. When participants are reading this phase, it helps to remind them that they would never have needed to develop the survival responses had the trauma not happened.

As Phase Four draws to a close, a certain peace tends to come over the individual. This differs, depending on how many sources of trauma the individual has, and whether or not another source of trauma has raised its ugly head. Internally, completing Phase Four succeeds in disassembling the second maze of emotions and loss which developed as a result of the survival responses.

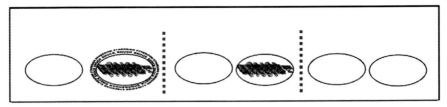

Figure 27: The Second Maze is Disassembled

At the same time, the repairs to the Existential Identity and the Operational Identity are being completed. As the mazes are disassembled, the person's values, beliefs, image, and reality become continuous once again.

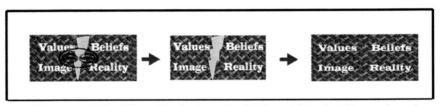

Figure 28: The Existential Identity is Repaired

The Operational component of the Identity is also repaired. First, the interaction between the restored Existential Identity and the Operational Identity resumes. Second, the interaction between the rational/cognitive and experiential attributes resumes. The result is that, just as before the trauma occurred, the person is well integrated again. The person's thinking and feeling work together to once again provide protection and manage the person's life. The following diagrams illustrate the changes that take place.

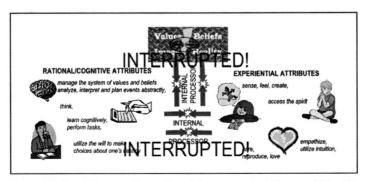

Figure 29: Post-Trauma Operational Component of Personal Identity

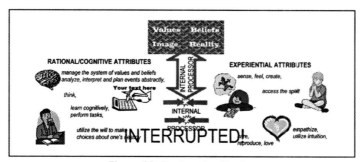

Figure 30: Restoration Begins

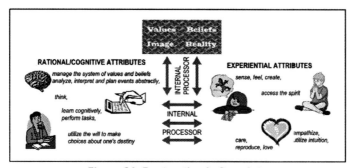

Figure 31: Restoration is Complete

Remember that complete restoration of a trauma survivor requires addressing *all* sources of trauma with *all* five phases of TRT. Survivors *will* experience great relief after completing only one out of three sources of trauma. However, the healing they experience when they have completed three out of three sources of trauma is *even better*!

Phases Five A and B summarize and complete the restoration. People react differently to Phase Five A. Some people are very emotional, while others experience little negative emotion when reading Five A. Five B, on the other hand, is very emotional in a good way. I try to bring new patients into the group during a Five B celebration, since it brings such hope to them.

When the trauma occurred, actual physiological changes took place in the brain of the trauma victim. The degree of change was determined by the intensity and frequency of the trauma. When restoration takes place, more physiological changes occur. These physiological changes take time, for the brain must develop new nerve pathways. This requires nothing of the person on a conscious level, other than cognitive focus through the structure of TRT. Just as the initial changes took place as a result of the trauma, these "good" changes take place automatically as the trauma is resolved. Sometimes the physiological changes lag behind the reading process. That means that a person will continue to see the shedding of survival responses even after finishing the five phases. Occasionally, with very long readings, the physiological changes seem to move faster than the reading process. Either way, completion of all the phases is necessary and will result in restoration of the trauma survivor. This does not mean that the person will be exactly like he or she was before the trauma occurred. Many other things have also changed in the person's life like age, surroundings, and interests. Change is a natural part of life. What will return, however, is the ability to deal with life without having the trauma as the main driving force in all interactions. The trauma survivor will be free to put God back into the appropriate place in his or her life.

[To view a more technical summary of what TRT accomplishes, including a neurological discussion of the effects of trauma and the resolution of trauma, please visit Etiotropic.org.]

Chapter Seven: Forgiveness and TRT

When I was in graduate school, I became depressed. Through prayer, God revealed to me that one of the contributing factors was my anger at a former boyfriend. After our dating in high school and off and on through college, he, for the third time, asked me to marry him. I decided that this time, I would say yes. After proposing, however, he stopped calling me and he would not return my calls. Several weeks later, he finally called and told me how morally superior he was to me and that he was marrying someone else. I was deeply wounded and angry. God revealed to me my lack of forgiveness two years later. I said to God, "Okay, I choose to obey you and forgive him, but I really feel like I need to talk to him and tell him how he hurt me. So if you will bring him across my path, then I will confront him." By then, I had no idea where he was. Well, God does not waste time. Two days later, I was driving home from graduate school in Atlanta, Georgia, on Interstate 85 North (a six-lane highway just counting the northbound side) during rush hour, and a guy in a car drove up next to me and started waving. I thought he was flirting and ignored him. He was persistent, and I finally recognized him as my former boyfriend. What were the chances of his seeing me on a six-lane highway with a zillion cars traveling at 60 miles an hour, let alone recognizing me, and wanting to wave me down? It had to be prearranged by God! He followed me off the highway and agreed to come right then to my house to talk. I expressed all of my hurt and anger, and he apologized sincerely. God had evidently also been dealing with him. He left, I cried, and I thanked God for the healing

I felt through forgiving that man. When we make the choice to forgive (an act of the will), it is amazing what God will do to help us along in our emotional healing.

For others affected by trauma, the experience of forgiveness may be more complicated than the one I have described and may take the assistance of someone outside of themselves who is experienced in working with trauma survivors. The process of forgiveness is the same for everyone, but—for trauma survivors—the overwhelming pain of thinking about the details of the trauma and acknowledging their losses frequently keeps them stuck. The shame of the trauma also keeps their focus on themselves and they may find themselves refusing to forgive out of a need for protection.

On the other hand, many people turn to forgiveness thinking that this will enable them to *avoid* dealing with the pain and loss of their experiences. Although spiritual maturity takes place through hard times, many well-meaning Christian people say that not dwelling on the past is showing a lot of faith in God. I disagree. I think that not processing past losses shows a lack of spiritual growth. When we are willing to go through the *process* of experiencing forgiveness on all levels—cognitive, emotional, spiritual and physical— we not only receive freedom but also our faith grows by leaps and bounds. Our faith is stretched as we believe that God will take us through the pain, and we stop trying to look for a way around it.

"Forgive and forget," "just let it go," "move on," and "don't dwell on the past" are all phrases heard by trauma victims from well-meaning, although misinformed, loved ones. As Christians, we are instructed by God to forgive those who sin against us and to love our enemies.

Matthew 6:12 "Forgive us our debts, as we also have forgiven our debtors. 14 For if you forgive men when they sin against you, your heavenly Father will also forgive you. 15 But if you do not forgive men their sins, your Father will not forgive your sins."

Ephesians 4:32 "Be kind and compassionate to one another, forgiving each other, just as in Christ God forgave you."

When it comes to trauma, forgiving can be a confusing task. Understanding what forgiveness is and the purpose of forgiveness are keys to experiencing true forgiveness. There are many reasons why God commands us to forgive.

- In 2 Corinthians 2:10-11 Paul wrote:

    "If you forgive anyone, I also forgive him. And what I have forgiven—if there was anything to forgive—I have forgiven in the sight of Christ for your sake, in order that Satan might not outwit us. For we are not unaware of his schemes."

    Satan uses unforgiveness to bring disharmony into the church as well as to the individual. Unforgiveness, whether it is trauma related or not, leaves an open door for evil spirits to come in and raise havoc.

- Just prior to the above passage, verses 5-8, Paul wrote:

    If anyone has caused grief, he has not so much grieved me as he has grieved all of you, to some extent—not to put it too severely. The punishment inflicted on him by the majority is sufficient for him. Now instead, you ought to forgive and comfort him, so that he will not be overwhelmed by excessive sorrow. I urge you, therefore, to reaffirm your love for him.

    Paul appears to be talking about a repentant believer in this passage. When others are unwilling to forgive a brother or sister, they may become depressed. This can lead to many other spiritual and emotional problems. Again, Satan will get a victory if we remain in unforgiveness.

- In Matthew 18:21 Peter asked Jesus how many times he should forgive someone who sinned against him. He then suggested what he thought was a very generous number—*seven* times. Jesus replied with *seventy seven times*, meaning that we should forgive an unlimited number of times. Verses 23-35 then record the following story which Jesus told Peter.

    Therefore, the kingdom of heaven is like a king who wanted to settle accounts with his servants. As he began the settlement, a man who owed him ten thousand talents was brought to him. Since he was not able to pay, the master ordered that he and his wife and his children and all that he had be sold to repay the debt. The servant fell on his knees before him. " Be patient with me,"' he begged, 'and I will pay back everything.' The servant's master took pity on him, canceled the debt and let him go. But when that servant went out, he found one of his fellow servants who owed him a hundred denarii. He grabbed him and began to choke him. 'Pay back what you owe me!' he demanded. His fellow servant fell to his knees and begged him, 'Be patient with me, and I will pay you back.' But he refused. Instead, he went off and had the man thrown into prison until he could pay the debt. When the other servants saw what had happened, they were greatly distressed and went and told their master everything that had happened. Then the master called the servant in. 'You wicked servant,' he said, 'I canceled all that debt of yours because you begged me to. Shouldn't you have had mercy on your fellow servant just as I had on you?' In anger his master turned him over to the jailers to be tortured until he should pay back all he owed. This is how my heavenly Father will treat each of you unless you forgive your brother from your heart."

God commands us to forgive others and to show gratitude for how we have been forgiven by Him. He did not have to forgive us, but out of His mercy He chose to let Jesus pay the debt and let us go free. When we forgive others, we are reflecting His way of extending mercy to them.

- The Scripture is clear and consistent. If we go on hating—not forgiving—then we are, at the least, confused and, at the most, lost. There is no qualification such as "but if you've been abused you don't have to forgive."

    I John 2:11 "But whoever hates his brother is in the darkness and walks around in the darkness; he does not know where he is going, because the darkness has blinded him."

If you are a trauma survivor, about this time you may be feeling guilty and telling yourself, *"See this is all my fault. I just have to forgive and go on with my life."* Or, you may be angry at me and at God saying, *"You make it sound so simple. You don't understand what I've been through!"* I urge you, **do not throw this book down now! Keep reading**. Read it all before jumping to those conclusions. Forgiveness is commanded, but Christ did not say it was "simple." There is more to it, or the book would end here.

Forgiveness Myths

Now let us look at what forgiveness is *not*. **Forgiveness is not forgetting**. God says that He remembers our sins no more. God knows everything. It is not so much that he *forgets* our sins as we forget what day our teeth were cleaned when we were 8 years old. Instead, He does not hold our sins against us any more. Even if God is able to forget in the way we forget, we are not God and we do not have that kind of control over our brains. Many trauma victims experience loss of memory around traumatic events. This is actually a survival response and not a sign of forgiveness. Lost memories are sometimes triggered by new events, and sometimes they are lost forever. Even after you have forgiven someone for sinning against you, you will remember that it took place. You will, however, think about it less and less. Also, the intensity of emotion connected with it will decrease.

Forgiveness is not minimizing the importance of the incident. When people apologize for hurting my feelings, I catch myself saying, "Oh, that's okay," even if it were not "okay." Abuse of *any* kind is *never* okay, but many people confuse their willingness to say "no big deal" with true forgiveness. Also, forgiving someone does not indicate that the abuse was not serious. When God forgives us, it is not because our sins were not serious, but rather because He is Gracious and Merciful. He *wants* to forgive us.

Forgiveness is not letting someone off the hook. Our continuing to hate someone because of his or her abuse does not punish or hurt only that person—it hurts all of us. Unlike God, when *we* forgive someone it benefits us as well as the other person. As long as we stay hatefully angry at others, we stay emotionally bound to them. When we focus on them, that is who we become *like*. The longer we hate, the more control they have over our lives. God instructs us to forgive, because He knows how it will benefit all of us. He also says that He will deal with the abuser.

> *Matthew 18:6-7 But if anyone causes one of these little ones who believe in me to sin, it would be better for him to have a large millstone hung around his neck and to be drowned in the depths of the sea. Woe to the world because of the things that cause people to sin! Such things must come, but woe to the man through whom they come!*

The abuser is still responsible for his or her actions. The consequence of the abuser's sin is death, the same as the consequence of the trauma survivor's sin.

Forgiveness does not necessarily mean reestablishing a relationship with someone. Remember the story I told at the beginning of this chapter about an ex-boyfriend? Reestablishing a relationship would have been very inappropriate in that case. There are a multitude of situations in which a person can find themselves when dealing with forgiving an abuser. Prayer and Godly counsel should always be sought before reestablishing a relationship that has already been severed. Continuing in an abusive relationship is not usually God's will for an individual, but each person must determine that for himself or herself. Remember what Christ said in Matthew 7:6

> *"Do not give dogs what is sacred; do not throw your pearls to pigs. If you do, they may trample them under their feet, and then turn and tear you to pieces."*

Wild pigs are wild pigs. They have always been wild pigs, and they will always be wild pigs. Even if you lay before them your most precious and valued possession, a string of beautiful pearls, they will follow their nature. They will trample them and attack you. Some people are like pigs. They do not value your precious forgiveness or you. Forgiving them is a command from God, but putting yourself in a position to be trampled upon is not wise and is not "love."

Forgiveness is not just a feeling. Forgiveness is a decision and an experience. We must decide out of our wills that we will forgive someone. That is an act of obedience to God. When we obey God, He blesses that decision and puts us in a position to experience forgiveness on an emotional level.

Forgiveness does not have to involve confrontation. If that were the case, everyone would have to look up his or her abuser; and if they were dead, you could not fulfill God's command. Each person should seek God and Godly counsel before ever confronting an abuser. Most abusers deny having done anything. Some even blame the person they abused. If you plan to continue or reestablish a relationship with the abuser, confrontation at some point may be necessary or unavoidable. Do not make a hasty decision about confrontation. As in the story I shared about myself, God will make it happen in His timing.

Forgiveness and the Cycle of Grief

For many people the first step is the *decision* to forgive. Others start into the process of resolution and are in the middle when confronted with the decision. Elizabeth Kubler Ross[19] is well known for identifying the stages of grief experienced by terminally ill people and their families. As a result of their multiple losses, trauma survivors go through these same stages of grief. The stages of grief are: shock, denial, anger turned inward, anger turned outward, acceptance of the pain, and resolution. I believe that forgiveness takes place, or is experienced, as a person moves through these stages. Let me emphasize that the term *stages* is used loosely. This process is not structured like the phases of TRT are structured. People move in and out and around and up and down before completing the grieving process. The use of the term *stages* is to emphasize that at certain times certain things are experienced more intensely than at other times. This process of grieving sometimes leaves a person wondering if there is something wrong with him or her. The use of *stages* is also to emphasize that it is normal to experience this variety of emotions, thoughts, and behavior.

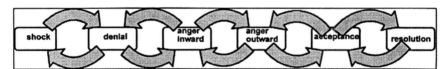

Figure 32: The Cycle of Grief.

The first stage is shock. In this stage a person is generally numb or dumbfounded about the event. He or she has difficulty believing that it actually happened. He or she may have memory loss around the event or may not recall it at all. When my youngest brother was in high school, he was hit by a car while walking into the school. He does not remember the incident or even driving to school that day. Graciously his brain has blocked out that painful memory, probably forever. Rape victims are often disoriented, confused, and show little emotion while being examined in emergency rooms.

The next stage is denial. In this stage the person has more recall of the event and may have a lot of emotion about the event, but he or she minimizes what occurred or how it affected him or how it currently impacts her life. Many people say, "Yes, I was sexually abused by my father, but I have a great relationship with him now and we just don't talk about it." Of course, they are in my office for severe depression, but that is not why they are depressed! Many Christians say, "Yes, my mom used to beat me and threaten to kill me, but I have forgiven her and she's a Christian now, so that can't be why I can't stop overeating and have these anger outbursts." Being saved does not take away all the effects of our's, and others', sin. In Romans 12:2 Paul said:

> *"Do not conform any longer to the pattern of this world, but be transformed by the renewing of your mind. Then you will be able to test and approve what God's will is—his good, pleasing and perfect will."*

Transformation is a *process* following salvation. Salvation *is* instantaneous.

The next two stages are the anger stages—anger turned inward and anger turned outward. Anger turned inward frequently occurs first, though a person moves around in the grief cycle in many directions before reaching resolution. Anger turned inward takes the form of self-blame, self-hate, taking responsibility for the abuse, disgust with self, etc.

This first "half" of the grief cycle is where many trauma survivors get "stuck." They flip back and forth between these first stages with no way of crossing over into "anger turned outward" and more empowerment. This is why trauma survivors are viewed as having such a "victim mentality" by those around them. Survival frequently means avoiding any anger at the perpetrator, or avoiding any feelings at all. While a person experiences many feelings, as described in previous chapters, the stages are named for the central experience of that stage. Moving through the stages is not like walking in and out of doors, either. They are not that cut and dried. One stage morphs into another. As a person moves through the grief stages, his or her emotions become more defined and more focused.

The anger-turned-outward stage is initially experienced as irritation, frustration, and annoyance, generally at everyone. Then it progresses into definable anger in general, or at all men, all women, all bosses, etc. Finally it becomes intense rage, even hatred, aimed specifically at the perpetrator. This progression must take place in order for the person to move successfully on to the next stage. Until the trauma survivor has experienced anger specifically at the perpetrator, he or she cannot move into acceptance of the pain.

Stop Treating Symptoms and Start Resolving Trauma!

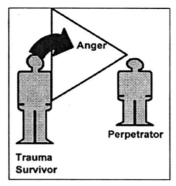

Figure 33: Anger Becomes More Focused On the Perpetrator As the Survivor Moves Through the Anger Stages.

For the trauma survivor, the "acceptance" stage means accepting the reality of the trauma, accepting the pain of the trauma and accepting that significant losses did occur. This stage is where true mourning takes place. A survivor must acknowledge the specific losses which occurred as a result of the trauma and as a result of his or her attempts to survive. Each of these losses must be mourned. While crying may take place throughout all of the stages, crying changes a little in this stage. When finished crying, a person will feel some relief and some release. Each mourning episode leaves behind a little more strength and determination. Now that the individual is consciously aware of the extent of the damage the perpetrator has caused, true forgiveness can take place. A person must complete this stage before true forgiveness can be *completed,* but forgiveness *must* take place before the grief cycle is ended in resolution.

The final stage is resolution. In this stage the trauma is put into perspective in one's life. The trauma is not forgotten, and the person still has feelings about it, although not as intense. It is not the defining incident in the person's life, however. Think of it as sitting in a library and reading a book. You have been sitting there reading that same book over and over again for years. All you can think of is that book. All you talk about are the characters in that book. The story and the characters are very alive and present to you. During resolution, you get up, walk to one of the many library shelves and put the book away. You remember where you put it, and you still think about it sometimes, but you leave it on the shelf. The characters are people you used to know. The story is in the past. You pick up another book and sit down at the table to read. God can now be the central focus of your life again. You will begin to write new books and fill up more shelves. (Hopefully action/adventure or romance and not murder mystery.)

Denice Adcock Colson

How do we get from knowing the scriptural instruction to forgive to "All I have to do is forgive?" This makes it sound so simple, so fast, so painless. Forgiveness is a process although at some point a conscious decision must be made. For some people the decision seems to come more readily, yet others believe that their best protection is to refuse to forgive. Forgiveness is a sacrifice of self, but the payoff far outweighs the cost. The payoff is freedom, peace of mind, a new life and forgiveness from God. Healing for trauma survivors involves forgiveness, for forgiveness is an integral part of the resolution process. It is not the entire process, however.

Chapter Eight: Marriage and Family Counseling During the Trauma Recovery Process

Many trauma survivors are brought into counseling through marital conflict. Because survival responses continue to follow a person throughout his or her life and affect every relationship, marital conflict is common. Sometimes the trauma is from the past and sometimes it is current. This will have some affect on the way marital counseling is conducted.

There are two basic principles in marriage counseling when one or both of the spouses are participating in a TRT process. First, the purpose of marriage and/or family counseling is to begin the re-establishment of communication. As noted in earlier chapters, the communication system has broken down in families directly affected by trauma. Communication can also break down in families indirectly affected by trauma, i.e. families where one member (usually adult) has past (usually childhood) unresolved trauma. That is why couples who are addiction free, abuse free, and currently trauma free can attend marriage enrichment activities and read wonderful marriage enrichment books yet still remain frustrated in their attempts to develop the intimacy they require. The repressed trauma is below the surface, maintaining itself in the unconscious mind of the trauma survivor and continuing to foster survival responses (defenses) that sabotage intimacy. While certain progress appears to be made, it is the old saying, "One step forward, two steps back." Couples become increasingly frustrated and may even reach the point of hopelessness unless they understand the necessity of resolving past traumas.

Note the emphasis on *begin* in the first principle. During the trauma recovery process, progress in marriage and family counseling will be *slow*. Expectations for the re-establishment of communication should be set realistically low. Initial communication-skills development should be limited to expression of feelings and moderate problem solving. Basic "Susan, what did you hear John say? Please repeat it word for word." is the kind of communication employed at this point. Couples need to be prepared to wait on the intimacy they so crave in their relationship. This leads us to the second principle.

The second principle is that individual TRT progress must take priority over marriage or family progress (except when a crisis requires immediate or protective action). In truth, individual TRT progress will directly determine the marital or family progress. There are a variety of possible scenarios to consider in families affected by trauma.

1. The trauma source is the husband (or wife) who is a perpetrator.

2. The trauma source is the husband's (or wife's) past. Neither are perpetrators.

3. The trauma source is one of the children (young adult, teenager, pre-teen) who is a perpetrator (usually actively pursuing drug and alcohol use).

4. The trauma source is the husband's (or wife's) source of employment (crisis manager).

5. The trauma source is an intangible affecting the family (natural disaster, death of a loved one, illness, etc).

In each of these scenarios, as the trauma goes unresolved, communication shuts down, trust is lost, enmeshment sets in and the family will spiral out of control. All but one of these scenarios may require the simultaneous application of individual TRT processes as well as sporadic marital or family counseling. The exception is scenario 3. In this case, the individuals comprising the couple have the same source of trauma. They will both be writing about their child. This can be done separately in individual processes, or as I have done it, with the couple together. The two people form their own mini-TRT group. Ideally, a group of couples would form, but with no more than 3 to 4 couples in a group.

The goals of the TRT couples or family counseling should be clear. These should include:

1. We are getting together to make sure we are all on the same page. Our plan is to save this family from complete destruction (assuming that is their goal). Restate the treatment plan, i.e., each person is completing his or her individual TRT, each is in phase ____. From here we go to _____. Remember, progress in couples' counseling will be slow.

2. Let us be patient.

3. What happened this week? Includes basic events that took place and any crises that need to be addressed.

4. Please do not talk about this with each other during the week. Only talk about it in here.

5. Do not try to solve or make any major decisions. Try to put them off until each person has at least completed Phase Two.

Each time I meet with the couple, I try to cover the above 5 areas. I may meet every two weeks, every month or only when necessary.

TRT Couples' Counseling With Addicts

There are some special interventions you can do early on when you are dealing with an addict in couples' counseling with TRT. Addiction may include alcohol, other drugs, gambling, spending, pornography or sex. If the addict is within his or her first 6 months of sobriety or abstinence, group participation in TRT is not allowed. Five to six months of sobriety should be required before a recovering addict can be placed in a TRT group. In the meantime, the addict is asked to make a comprehensive list of all of his or her use episodes. He or she reads this list to the counselor or the substance abuse group members. The spouse also makes a list of all of the addict's use episodes of which he or she is aware. This is a list, not full TRT Phase One writings. It may be long and it may take a couple of weeks to write. Each episode is summarized on one or two lines of notebook paper. If other family members are going to participate, they also make a list of the addict's use episodes of which they are aware. When everyone is finished, you schedule a family session. Ideally, the addict will read his or her list in group or to the counselor 24-48 hours prior to the family session. In the family session, the addict is coached that he or she is not allowed to say anything until everyone has finished reading. He or she must sit and listen to everything without challenging, denying or in any way rebuffing the readers. The only thing he or she is allowed to say after everyone has finished is, "I'm sorry". That is all. The addict should know that, should he or she try to say anything else, the session will end and he or she will be removed. During the session, you start with the youngest child, if children are participating, and move to the oldest. The spouse is last. The children are removed before the spouse reads. Hopefully, the spouse and children will feel like they are being heard by the addict for the very first time. Hopefully, this will also lead to a sense of brokenness in the addict. To be clear, the addict does not read his or her list to any family members. There will be things on there of which no one else is aware. Sharing these things *will not help* the healing process.

Counseling with Couples When the Trauma is in the Past

Frequently, a woman comes to counseling alone and the most pressing trauma truly is in the past. Her husband is not a perpetrator; he may have his problems but is generally supportive of her getting help for unresolved trauma. In this case I encourage the client to bring her husband in with her after she has committed to the process. It is important to explain to the non-participating spouse what he can expect as his wife moves through the phases. He has, of course, been affected by the survival responses she has developed. He may be the brunt of some more before it is over. Warning him and supporting him as he supports her is very important.

More Advanced Marriage Counseling

One of the most helpful books I have used in TRT couples counseling is *The Five Love Languages*, by Gary Chapman. I have used this early on, just to try to settle things down as we went through the TRT process. Getting traumatized couples to read it is very difficult, however. Summarizing the concepts and helping them identify their love languages in a session is most effective. Again, do not set expectations too high in the beginning.

As the couple completes their individual Phase Two TRT processes, they are ready for the marriage counseling to begin to move forward. What I have found is that the couple needs less marriage counseling as they advance. However, there are a lot of good tools and reading materials to educate them on healthy relationships. I would still stay away from behavioral interventions that may challenge their survival responses, though. For example, I was supervising a female minister who was working with a female client while another minister was working with her husband. The minister was told by a few other staff members that this client was going around the church telling different people what her husband had done. They wanted her to stop because it made things uncomfortable for many people. Dutifully, she kindly confronted the client in an individual session, tactfully telling her that this information was going around the church and might not look good for her. The client missed the next two group sessions. When my supervisee began telling me about this incident, I caught my breath. "Oh no," I thought. I explained that the client was using a survival response that helped her survive the humiliation she experienced at home while her husband was experiencing so much popularity at church. By confronting the survival behavior, which may or may not have been appropriate, the minister had helped to further repress the trauma, created shame for the survivor and really angered her. My recommendation was to go to her and honestly apologize. Also, she should explain exactly what happened. This is what occurs when we mix behavioral techniques, however well intended, with TRT when the etiology has not been fully reversed.

Dr. Gary Smalley, in his book *Making Love Last Forever*,[20] points out that there are many ways to make a marriage work. People do a lot of things, based on their circumstances and their personalities, to make sure they stay married and stay in love. However, he says, there are only four basic ways to ruin a marriage.

They include:

1. Withdrawing during an argument.

2. Escalating the argument—getting louder, meaner, more aggressive.

3. Invalidating your mate's feelings.

4. Harboring false beliefs or false assumptions about your mate's feelings.

I agree with Dr. Smalley (one of my favorite writers and speakers) that these are all very destructive to marriages. However, these are also all *very common* survival responses in traumatized couples. Suggesting to a non-traumatized couple that they change these behaviors is appropriate and very helpful. Traumatized couples will take this information and do two things with it. The perpetrator will use it to further abuse, blame and scapegoat the victim. The victim will use it to further repress the trauma and support the projection of the perpetrator. That is why so many counselors and couples get so frustrated. They consume all of this wonderful information but cannot seem to apply it. They get increasingly agitated, blaming each other, until finally they reach the state of hopelessness.

A couple described the following scenario, in which all four of the previous warning factors were present. While they were getting into bed, he returned her kiss half-heartedly. She asked, "What's wrong? Are you mad at me for something?" He laid there silently for a few seconds, contemplating whether or not he wanted to get into the conversation. Finally he said, "yes" and described a time earlier when she had spoken to him in a way that hurt his feelings. She became angry because he waited so long to bring it up and then brought it up while they were in bed (3,4). Also, he was lying down as he talked and bringing it up in the "sanctuary" of the bedroom. She left the room to sit in the front room (1). When he did not follow her, she got angrier. She came back into the bedroom and said she was going to the grocery store (1,2,4). When she returned home an hour or so later, he was asleep. She became so angry that she woke him up, told him to take extra clothes to work tomorrow, and told him to find some other place to stay because she wanted a divorce (2, 3, and 4). They argued for several hours, and then argued some more in my office. In the therapy session, she continued saying that he was just like her ex-husband, that she would not allow herself to be hurt again like that, and that she would get a divorce if necessary (2, 3, and 4). She was currently writing about her ex-husband in TRT group. She had written stories of horrible abuse about her ex-husband including rapes, beatings, threats with guns, and abandonment. When I stated that her current husband was nothing like her former husband, she became furious with *me*. I had pushed on one of her survival responses.

Marital counseling while doing TRT can be tricky. You must tread softly, move slowly and have reasonable expectations. Assuring clients that they are normal and that very slow progress should be expected takes the pressure off, and hopefully, keeps them from going down the path of hopelessness. Eventually, the relationship can come together in a remarkable way. Remember that the focus is on completing the individual TRT, and as clients see themselves making progress, the pressure on the marriage will get better.

Chapter Nine: Using TRT with Adolescents and Children

When conducting training for ETM Certification, I am always asked, "Can you use TRT with children or adolescents?" My answer is "Yes" and "No." Yes, you can use the same five-phase process with children and adolescents that you use with adults. No, you cannot use it exactly the same all the time. It depends. In this chapter I will explore some of the creative ways I have successfully used TRT with various age groups.

Children

Phases Three and Four are usually not necessary with children but can be done in an abbreviated verbal form if absolutely necessary. I would only use it with older ones. When working with children, you may be able to use the normal structured incident writing of Phase One, depending upon the age and skills level of the child. However, you may need to either do the work verbally or have the child dictate to you. The Phase work, whether verbal or written, should be done in the counseling session and mixed with other counseling formats. For example, you may start with some free-play therapy, move to writing and reading, then end with coloring or drawing. If the child is not able or inclined to read or write, you can use drawings and story telling for Phase One. You can also use dolls for telling stories.

One of my favorite techniques is using photo albums. This is especially helpful in dealing with the death of a parent. You can have them bring in photo albums already made at home or make one in the office. They can tell you stories about the pictures and you can write them down, record them, or just listen and respond. At the point in the process when you ask, "What are you feeling?" they may need more help identifying feelings. Having them point to a feeling word chart with faces on it can help. You must also give feedback in words they understand.

The Phase Two Matrix can be done verbally or in writing. If done in writing, the child will most likely need a lot of assistance in filling in the columns. Verbally following the structure seems to work just as well with children as writing. You can also do a combination, filling it out for them as you talk.

Phase Five A can also be done verbally in an abbreviated form. Phase Five B can be done in the counseling session or as a project completed at home with a parent's assistance prior to the counseling session. This again depends on the child's age and motivation level.

The most important thing when doing TRT with children is following the structure of the five phases, resolving trauma in the order in which it developed, and avoiding focusing on symptoms. Since they have much more elasticity in their neurons, trauma reversal can be much quicker with children than with adults.

Adolescents

Teenagers provide challenges of their own in therapy, regardless of the approach you use. Having used a variety of techniques in a variety of settings, however, I have been surprised at the receptivity of teens to TRT. Perhaps it reminds them of schoolwork, and since it involves concrete activities, they seem to understand more of what is expected of them. Of course, when it comes to resolving trauma and actually getting something accomplished other than play, it stands head and shoulders above all other techniques. As with children, TRT is not the only thing done in the fifty-minute therapy session with adolescents. Teens are very "here and now;" last week is way in the past for them. Joining with them first is very important. Getting to know some of the things they like and dislike, talking about movies or music, boyfriends or girlfriends, school, sports and other interests is always important.

I try to stress to adolescents that I am not there to try to change them, make them better people, or even to make them behave. My job is to help them resolve the trauma they have experienced. I praise them for their writing efforts, for their reading in group or individual sessions, and for allowing me or others to see them cry. While I acknowledge positive changes outside of the session, I try to avoid praising them too much for that since I do not want to change the focus from resolving the trauma to changing the symptoms.

My personal preference is to start in family therapy with as many members as possible or appropriate, including siblings if they are old enough. Here I collect as much information and history as possible. Then I will usually dismiss the rest of the family and meet with the adolescent who is the identified patient. By this time I will usually have some idea of sources of trauma and will explore them further to get details they may not have been comfortable sharing in front of their parents. Of course, I always explain the limits of confidentiality before asking for disclosures. If time allows, I will then meet with the parents separately. I will explain my plan for treatment and more about trauma and how TRT works. I will offer a handout or book about TRT and ask them to think about whether they want to pursue this type of treatment for their teen or for the entire family.

The five-phase process of TRT with adolescents is the same as with adults. However, I never expect teens to do their writing at home; we always do it during the session. I explain to them what I want them to do, set them up with paper and a pen, then sit back and wait. Usually their biggest concern is that I might stare at them. I review their writings, just as with adults, and explain the changes I make. Then I have them read using the same structure as adults. Usually, I see little emotion with teens during the first several sessions and sometimes through the entire process. What I do see, however, is a reduction in survival responses at home and increased trust in the counseling relationship.

Phase Two is done just like Phase One: explain then sit back and wait, review and read. If they are necessary, Phases Three, Four and Five A are also completed in the same manner. These phases are more frequently necessary with teens than with children, but less so than with adults. Since teens are often brought into counseling because they are acting out, Phases Four and Five are frequently necessary.

Denice Adcock Colson

Adolescents in Traumatized Families

It is actually rare that I personally treat an adolescent for trauma without also treating at least the parents. Much of the time adolescents are the identified patients in traumatized families. Frequently, I uncover alcohol abuse or even addiction in one of the parents in the first or second session. This can be tricky when the parent wants the child fixed but is unwilling to change himself or herself. In one case the parents actually sent a previously drug-abusing teenager to counseling by way of a teenage friend with $90 cash in her pocket to pay the counseling fee. I insisted that our next visit would be a family session. In that meeting I confirmed that what the teen had said was true; her father was an alcoholic. Selling alcohol was his business and he made a lot of money doing it. Sobriety was, according to him, impossible. The parents desperately wanted to send the teenager to see me but were unwilling to participate in any other way. Even the wife/ mother was not willing to participate. I felt I had no choice but to refuse to see the teenager, given the liability issues. That was a very hard decision, since I did feel a lot of compassion for the teenager. Other counselors may have continued to see the teen, hoping at least to help her. Since my approach would have been TRT, I knew that as she worked on her own drug use and on her father's addiction, she would get more assertive and thus cause more problems for the family. I would be forcing her between a proverbial rock and a hard place. This type of stress is very difficult for an adult to handle, let alone a teenager. She had to continue to live with the perpetrator for survival. Since no physical or sexual abuse was going on, I had to hope that the mother would feel increased stress and eventually seek help for the whole family.

Often I will see teens who are really good kids—no drugs, alcohol or promiscuous sexual activity—but who are having severe difficulty in school and lots of conflict with their parents. As a TRT counselor, you must always look for trauma, not necessarily as you would define it, but trauma as it would be to a teenager. In otherwise calm families, a parent who has temper problems can be trauma. There may not be any name calling or hitting, just screaming. I have found that a five-phase process with teens like this does wonders. They like the structure and feel like they are finally heard. Family sessions, to get to the problems behind the screaming, can be done concurrently and may lead to more TRT with the parents for past trauma in their lives.

You must also keep an eye out for things that are *not* done as well as things that *are* done, like a parent who is a workaholic and does not attend recitals, parties, etc. It can be an estranged parent who does not pursue an ongoing relationship with his or her child—not visiting, not sending birthday cards or gifts, not calling, etc. Applying TRT can be confusing for the counselor since you must have the teenager write about things that *did not* happen, rather than things that *did* happen. Here is an example: "It was May 30, 2002. I was with my mom and John and my step-dad Bill. We went out to eat for my 15th birthday. You didn't call or send a birthday card or a gift. I felt forgotten, hurt and lonely. When I called and left a message at your house, you never called back. I felt rejected, unloved and abandoned." These incidents can have great impact on teens and children.

When at least one parent is willing to participate and the perpetrator is the other parent, I see the teen separately, using the same five-phase process. It can get expensive, so often I will divide a fifty-minute session in half, seeing the teen and maybe a sibling or parent for the other half.

Working with the Parents of Abusive Adolescents and Young Adults

When the teenager is the perpetrator, for example actively using drugs or alcohol, acting out physically or sexually, intervening with the parents can be the most effective intervention. The teen will pick one of the parents to do most of their projecting onto and an enmeshed relationship will form. This may rotate between parents and even other siblings. When one of the parents is NOT a perpetrator, I will immediately start the parents into TRT's five-phase process. This can be done individually, but I prefer to treat the parents together as a couple. They form their own little group. You can even put a group of parents together, all writing about their teens or young adults. This works well as outpatient counseling to support your treatment of addicted teens in a residential or inpatient setting.

The addicted teen should have five to six months of sobriety before starting the actual five-phase TRT process. During that time, you should use more traditional, supportive counseling as well as some type of 12 Step process to focus on sobriety. At the same time, the parents and possibly other siblings are working on their TRT and will move from accepting the teen's projection to setting limits without the counselor's having to "teach" limits and risk alienating the family.

Although I started working with teens in 1982, the beginning of my counseling career, I have found working with teens to be much more enjoyable and satisfying since I started using TRT. I get to avoid most types of conflict with them, do not have to take on a parental role, and even get to look like a hero sometimes. As a TRT counselor, you have to keep from getting a big head. It is not because you are so wonderful that they get better, but rather it is because the process works! All you have to do is apply it correctly and follow the structure.

Chapter Ten: Addiction as a Perpetrator

It is obvious to most people how living with an addict is trauma—the drunkenness, unpredictability, lying, stealing, cheating, and emotional, if not physical, absence. No other theory that I am currently aware of, however, addresses the trauma the addiction creates for the addicts *themselves*. Collins and Carson initially used TRT with recovering addicts and their families and in that environment became aware of the broad application of TRT. Many of the symptoms that sober addicts describe—such as rages, flashbacks, and nightmares—have been interpreted by addictions' counselors as cravings and relapse warnings. What if, however, they are symptoms of post-traumatic stress? Many addictions' counselors have been indoctrinated by the psychoanalytic model that says that adult dysfunctional behavior is the result of maladaptive or destructive relationships during the addict's childhood with the parents. Therefore, when thinking about trauma, they skip right over the actual addiction and look at previous—before they started using—trauma which may have led the person to choose addiction as a way to cope or manage negative feelings. When this is done, the trauma from the addiction is minimized and repressed further. The survivor never gets the real picture of the addiction as a perpetrator.

An addictive substance can be likened to a "date rapist." You go out with someone you do not know well, but other people you know have been out with the person before and had no problems. You want to get to know the person, so you talk, get comfortable, maybe even move a little closer. As you are spending time together, however, the person suddenly changes. He or she begins to force you or coerce you into doing things you had not planned to do and that you believe are wrong. Survival for you may mean fighting back or giving in. Either way, your life is changed forever. I have worked with many addicts, and none of them claims to have started out *wanting* to become an addict. No one has said, "When I was growing up, I wanted to be a cocaine addict!" People start using addictive substances for various reasons. Some include:

"Its fun; it helps me to relax."

"It helps me to forget about my problems for a while."

"All my friends were doing it, and I wanted to feel a part of the gang."

"I was curious about what it felt like to get high."

"I wanted to do anything my parents said I couldn't do."

As they *play* with the substance, something happens. Chemical reactions take place in the person's body that he or she is unaware of and over which he or she has no control. While losing control is the goal of getting high for most people, they think it stops when the substance wears off. What they are not aware of are the changes that have taken place in their nervous systems and in the biochemical makeup of their bodies. A person makes a choice about what he or she puts into his or her body; but once the substance is in the body, he or she has few if any choices left except to let it run its course.

It is ridiculous to expect someone to control himself or herself while high or to "hold his liquor." Consider this analogy. A salesman tells you there is a new diet that is guaranteed to work. First he takes your $100. Then he tells you to get your favorite food, say chocolate cake, and eat as much of it as you want. After eating the cake, you must concentrate and say to the cake, "Cake, I want you to pass through my body leaving only the good, nutritious things behind. I want all the fat and calories to pass right on through and cause no weight gain or increased insulin levels in my body." The salesman tells you that if you concentrate hard enough you can eat cakes until you are overly stuffed, every day of the week, and never gain any weight. Will you ask for the $100 back or follow the diet plan? Just as it is ridiculous to expect that diet plan to work, it is ridiculous to expect someone to control himself or herself while high or to "hold his or her liquor."

Alcohol and drugs are poisons. Taken in certain amounts they are toxic and even fatal. Many drugs, including alcohol, have medicinal purposes when taken in prescribed doses. Many street drugs were developed for medicinal purposes but have been found to have too many negative side effects or just did not do what they were supposed to do. Now they have no medicinal purpose—they are just toxic. The side effects of the toxicity are what people call a "high." Thus, they walk a fine line between dying and feeling good. The effect of the drugs is to actually alter their brain chemistry, sometimes permanently, and therefore the way they think, act, and perceive reality. The personality can be drastically altered with continued use of alcohol and/or drugs. Therefore, a person will do and say things under the influence and, with continued use, not under the influence that he or she would otherwise not do or say. The "toxic behavior" contradicts his or her underlying values, beliefs, image, and reality. The same four patterns of trauma occur for the addict as for the non-addicted trauma victim.

Take George for example. George was young, handsome and going places. Unfortunately he drank beer and hard liquor heavily. He also smoked pot, snorted cocaine, and played with several other drugs. He loved his wife and believed that he should treat her with respect. One night she went out with some friends after work and came home a little late. George drank and snorted coke until she came home. When she came through the door smiling, he erupted into a rage. He screamed at her, calling her a bitch, then grabbed her and threw her on the bed. He slapped her in the face several times then stormed out of the house. He saw that she looked terrified and that her mouth was bleeding. To the people who can relate to George's wife, this incident will bring rage and hurt. To those who can relate to George, this incident will bring feelings of understanding, and probably embarrassment and shame. Let us look at how the four patterns of trauma apply to this incident.

1. George's toxic behavior—screaming at his wife, calling her names, hitting her, leaving her bleeding on the bed while he stormed out—contradicted his values, beliefs, image and reality. George believed that he should love his wife and treat her with respect. He believed that hitting people was wrong. (He had decided as a

child that he would never hit his wife like he saw his father hit his mother.)

2. The contradictions resulted in loss. George lost self-esteem, self-control, self-confidence, the image of himself as a good husband, relationship with his wife, intimacy, masculinity, relationship with God, love from his wife, etc. These losses were repressed.

3. Survival responses developed. George began to think, "She deserves what she gets when she aggravates me like that!" He began to stay out later. He came home later and pretended nothing ever happened. He lied to some friends who asked why his wife had a bruised face. He drank and used drugs even more.

4. These survival responses also contradicted George's beliefs about what he should be doing. He experienced more losses of self-esteem, self-confidence, self-control, self-image, his image of his wife, relationships with friends, trust from his wife and friends, trust in his wife, relationship with God, etc. These losses were also repressed.

The same maze of emotional circuitry and loss develops for the addict as for the non-addicted trauma victim. Even when the initial trauma ends, i.e., the addict gets sober, the survival responses will continue and even increase until the trauma is resolved. "Dry drunk" is the phrase commonly used for this chaotic and doomed state of being. Most recovering addicts are told that sobriety is all they need. "Just follow the 12 Steps." Sometimes counseling or family therapy is recommended. The trauma work is usually focused on the "true victims," the family of the addict, or on trauma prior to the addiction. "Switching addictions" often occurs for recovering addicts. They may begin to smoke cigarettes, drink caffeine excessively, work obsessively, or any other number of survival responses. In fact, using alcohol and drugs frequently starts out as a survival response related to past trauma. It becomes a trauma in itself due to the nature of the substances and their addictive qualities.

Substance abuse and violence frequently go together, but not all addicts become violent. This lack of violence is often pointed out by trauma survivors and addicts as evidence that they are not addicted. Therefore, let us apply the four stages in the development of trauma to a non-violent addict.

Michael came to see me with his wife and two children. Their 13-year-old son was having difficulty in school and acting out at home. As I interviewed the family, it became apparent to me that Michael had a drinking problem. Nevertheless, the family totally denied that his drinking was a problem for them or for him. Michael came home from work, took his dinner into the bedroom to eat in front of his television, (and to drink scotch), then sat in his armchair drinking scotch until he passed out. His wife would pick up his glass, cover him with a blanket and go to bed without him. This happened *every* night. On weekends he spent some time around the house, then started drinking around 4 p.m. and drank until he passed out in his chair. On Sundays he went to church with the family for morning services. He repeated the same drinking behavior in the evenings. Michael was 38 years old. The family was convinced that because he was not violent, went to work everyday and to church on Sundays that his drinking could not possibly be a problem. As further evidence, they pointed out that he was a deacon in the church. Let us break down the four patterns of trauma for both Michael and the family.

1. Michael's toxic behavior, (withdrawing from his family, not sleeping with his wife, drinking until he passed out) contradicted his values and beliefs about what he should be doing. He believed he should be interacting with his wife, playing with his children, helping out around the house, and sleeping with his wife.

2. The contradictions resulted in loss. Michael lost self-esteem, time with his family, intimacy with his wife, respect from his family, years of his life, self-respect, etc. These losses were then repressed.

3. The repressed losses fostered survival responses. Michael lied to himself about what he wanted out of life, and he lied to his family about how satisfied he was. He denied he had a drinking problem, and he drank more.

4. The survival responses also contradicted Michael's values and beliefs about what he should be doing. He believed that a real man dealt with problems head on, that it was a sin to lie, and that drunkenness was a sin. These contradictions resulted in more loss, and those losses were also repressed.

Now let us look at how the trauma developed for Michael's 13-year-old son Mark.

1. Mark's father's toxic behavior (sitting in his room to eat, not interacting with Mark, not showing authority in the family) contradicted Mark's values and beliefs about what a father should do and be. Mark believed that fathers should spend time playing or working with their sons. He believed that fathers should not get drunk, that men worked around the house, took care of the yard, fixed things, etc. He was taught that drugs were wrong, that lying was wrong, and that laziness was wrong.

2. These contradictions resulted in loss. Mark lost respect for his father, a male role model, time with his dad, the opportunity to learn skills in home maintenance, the opportunity to have his dad at his baseball games, etc. These losses were repressed.

3. The repressed loss fostered survival responses. Mark began to avoid doing his homework. Instead, he would stay away from the house alone or with friends. He stopped trying to be polite to his teachers and he withdrew from his friends at school. He would not bring friends to his house for fear they would see his father, he refused to do anything with his father on the weekends, and he talked back to both his parents.

4. These survival responses also contradicted Mark's values and beliefs about what he should be doing. He believed that he should respect his father and mother. He believed he should get good grades, should hang out with his friends, and should have friends to his house. These contradictions resulted in more loss and the additional losses were also repressed.

Addiction, whether there is violence, verbal abuse, or withdrawal, is trauma for both the addict and the loved ones. The resolution process for the recovering addict is basically the same as for the non-addicted trauma victim. The writing is done in first person rather than second person, and information about what and how much of the alcohol/drugs were used is included. The recovering addict must maintain at least six months of sobriety before beginning a group experience of TRT. This gives time for his or her body to rid itself of most of the toxins, depending on what and how much he or she was using. Also, the nervous system has a chance to recover and get back to somewhat normal functioning. The individual will begin to experience and identify feelings again and may even experience empathy for others. Usually the empathy is for other recovering addicts and not for their traumatized spouses. Empathy for their families *will* come *if* they continue in TRT.

Outpatient TRT groups for recovering addicts are much more difficult to develop than groups for non-recovering victims. For one thing, before an addict can participate in the five-phase therapeutic process of TRT group, he or she must remain sober for six months. The addict must also begin to show some ability to empathize with another human being. Recovering addicts and non-addicts are never mixed in the same group, in order to insure that the focus remains on the trauma and does not switch to other group members.

During the first six months, while the focus is on sobriety, pre-TRT activities can take place. The survivor can be educated as to the effects of trauma on his or her life, he or she can participate in occasional family or couples therapy, and he or she can make a trauma incident list.

The trauma incident list will focus only on the addiction. The survivor is asked to make a list of all incidents of using drugs or alcohol that he or she can remember. For addicts with much longevity, this is best done in time *periods*. For example, starting with the first time he used and continuing in chronological order, the list may look something like this:

I was 16 and took some vodka from my dad's liquor cabinet. A friend and I drank in the back yard. I threw up and my parents thought I had the flu.

I drank off and on until I was 17, then I smoked pot for the first time after a football game with some friends. I got really stoned and couldn't find my car to go home. It scared me so bad I didn't use drugs again until I was in college.

I drank a fifth of vodka at a graduation party when I was 18. I stripped to my underwear and danced on stage until someone pulled me off. I passed out and threw up all over myself. My girlfriend never spoke to me again.

In college I started smoking pot again....

On my first job, I stayed sober for six months then started drinking after work with buddies.

When I was 25 I started using cocaine....

When I was 27 I went to rehab for the first time...

This list does not have to have great detail, and it is not supposed to be written using the five rules for writing used in Phase One. It should be as extensive as possible, but each incident or group of incidents will be briefly described. This list may take weeks for the survivor to complete, but it should be reviewed with the counselor on a weekly basis to keep the focus on moving toward doing TRT. Once it is completed, there are a couple of options for reading it. Ideally it would be read in a Chemical Dependency pre-TRT group. Otherwise, it should be read in an individual session with the counselor.

Another option for the list reading is to coordinate it with any ongoing marital or family therapy. This would mean that, as the addict survivor is writing his/her list, the family members are also making lists. Their lists would include any and all incidents they recall about the addict's using behavior and any abusive or traumatic incidents. Their lists would also be extensive but brief descriptions and would be read to the addict in a structured family session. This intervention is described in more detail in the chapter on Marriage and Family Counseling During the TRT Process.

When the addict is nearing 5-6 months of sobriety and begins to show some ability to empathize with others, he or she is ready to transition into the TRT group. He or she can use his or her list to begin writing fully developed incidents and practice reading them in individual sessions before moving to group. The rest of the process is the same as for non-addicted TRT participants. If an addict survivor relapses, he or she is moved to individual counseling temporarily and then back to group, if he or she returns to sobriety.

Other types of addictions, including sex/pornography addiction, can also benefit from the application of TRT's five phases. The modifications are the same as for alcohol/drug addiction. A full six months of sobriety is not required, however. We start with behavioral intervention to gain some sobriety, list writing and reading, and then begin the five-phase process. The same family list-writing intervention can be used as with alcohol/drug addiction survivors. A typical sex/pornography addiction Phase One incident may sound like this:

It was December of 2001. I was at home while my wife took the kids to a church Christmas party. I got on the computer right after they left and started surfing for porn. I felt excited but guilty. I looked at porn sites of women and men having sex and masturbated. I spent the entire two hours they were gone on the computer. When they got home I felt ashamed and guilty. I said I felt sick and went to bed early to avoid my wife. The next day I pretended nothing had happened.

Anorexia and Bulimia can also benefit from the application of TRT's five phases. A typical Phase One incident may sound like this:

It was January 2000. I felt bored and extremely anxious. I went to the drive-thru windows of McDonald's, Kentucky Fried Chicken and Krispy-Kreme Donuts. I ate a Big Mac, large fries, chocolate shake, two chicken thighs, a drum stick, a biscuit, mashed potatoes with gravy, and a dozen chocolate glazed donuts as fast as I could. I felt stuffed and sick. I went into the bathroom and threw up. I felt calmer. I also felt disgusted, frustrated, fat, ugly, ashamed, embarrassed and hopeless.

There are some difficulties when doing outpatient TRT with addicts. Recovering addicts rarely report for outpatient therapy to address their addiction, unless they are moved directly from intensive day treatment into an existing group. Most often recovering or active addicts come in for marital counseling, forced by their spouses or possibly their parents. With addicts, the survival responses of denial and blaming are *so* strong, and frequently supported by their surrounding recovery groups and possibly even counselors, that breaking through the synergism is very difficult. "Hitting bottom" is almost always necessary. Most recovering addicts have more than one source of trauma; therefore, everything discussed in the section titled "Multiple Sources of Trauma" applies to them. And, even if the trauma has stopped—they are no longer actively using—the cycle of projection and counter projection still continues with the spouse unless the spouse has entered TRT and progressed through Phase Two. Therefore, the spouse is frequently enabling the recovering addict to avoid the TRT work. Addiction usually lasts for years, once it has started. The repressed loss and emotion is overwhelming. Recovering addicts are not used to feelings and are used to medicating their feelings. They become overwhelmed with emotion very easily and terrified of feelings driving them into using again. This belief is often reinforced by recovery programs which tell participants that anger, sadness, and other grief emotions are symptoms of relapse and therefore to be avoided. However, addicts can successfully make it through the five-phase TRT process. When they do, they are very clear about what the addiction has stolen from them and their families and have difficulty seeing substances as friends ever again.

A common activity in substance abuse treatment is the writing of a life story. This *begins* the identification of the trauma; but if it stops there, it is simply evoking emotion and that is not enough to resolve trauma. It is my belief that, if Trauma Resolution became an established part of substance abuse treatment, the results could be astonishing. I believe that relapse rates would decrease dramatically; people would truly change and not just get sober. Families would stay together, and abuse would stop for good. It is not enough to just address the trauma of the family members of a recovering addict. The trauma experienced by the addicts from their own addiction must also be addressed.

Chapter Eleven: ETM for Crisis Management Personnel and Organizations

In 1993 or 1994 I received a referral from my former pastor. A couple had lost their little baby girl to SIDS. The mother was pleased one morning when the baby slept later than she ever had before, but, when she went to check on her, she was lying dead in her crib. The mother called 911 and the fire department came. Her husband made it home just as the lead fire fighter was removing the baby's body from the home. They were devastated! I took them through the short-form and (unbelievably) in 3 sessions they were ready to move on. They created their own 5B, a beautiful and touching poem in tribute to the short life of their lovely baby.

Shortly after their last visit, I received another referral from a different referral source. As the client, a fire fighter, sat in front of me and described the problem, I realized the story sounded very familiar. Suddenly it dawned on me that this was the fire fighter who had been required to remove the lifeless body of the infant belonging to the couple I had just finished seeing. I felt a mixture of intrigue and compassion. What fate that both parties had been referred to me from separate sources! I was able to get a multi-dimensional view of what took place.

He described having many PTS symptoms following that particular call. He had a child almost a year older than the infant, but his baby was still sleeping in a crib. He had become obsessed with the well being of his child. He had begun to have difficulty sleeping, had become extremely irritable, and was experiencing marital strife. He had ruminating thoughts, going over and over the experience of removing the child from her crib. I explained to him the four phases in the development of Trauma, how trauma was retained in the existential identity, and why crisis managers were different from non-crisis managers. He identified clearly with the theory and we began the short form of TRT. After 2 or three sessions, he no longer needed me for that particular trauma incident.

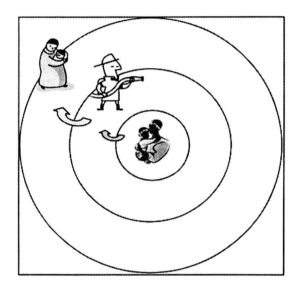

Figure 34 - The Ripple Effect

Let us get an over-all picture of this incident. The trauma occurred in the family, and it was then "passed" to the fire fighter. We call this the "Ripple Affect." Trauma is rarely isolated, but similar to dropping a pebble into a pond, the ripples continue outward, affecting more and more people. The further out in the ripple a person is, the less intense the affect of the trauma will be, at least initially. As you may then imagine, my story does not end there.

Approximately one year later, my husband and I had our first baby, a beautiful little girl named Rebecca. Following my C-section, I had to sleep on the downstairs sofa because I could not climb the stairs to our bedroom. We put Rebecca in a cradle right next to the sofa and my husband slept upstairs. It had been a year since I had treated both the couple who had lost their baby to SIDS and the fire fighter who had made the call. I was not even on the scene; I heard the entire story second-hand, yet, I could not get it out of my mind. Lying there on that couch, trying to sleep, I could see the entire scenario happening in my head, flashing before my eyes. I could not sleep, I cried, and I was terrified! I listened to every sound the baby made. Unfortunately, she was born with a loose piece of cartilage (according to the doctor) and she made a little rattling sound when she breathed. I was sure she was dying! Even when she was napping, I had to be right next to her. It was extremely painful. All I could think about was, "What if my baby dies the same way?!!" Finally, I had enough understanding to figure out what was happening to me. Up until this point I had not talked about it to anyone. I finally "broke down" and told my husband. He led me through a modified short-form of TRT and the obsessing stopped. Let me clearly state that he took me through it several times over a couple of days, but the painful obsessing and the terror stopped. (Fortunately, my husband had also been through the training several years earlier, but that is a different story.) I emphasize "broke down," because that is exactly the feeling a Crisis Manager frequently has before he or she can let it out. Just talking about it is very painful. It also violates some professional defense mechanisms of "This is my job. I am good at it and I am tough. I can handle it!" Breaking down is interpreted as a sign of weakness or inadequacy.

The ripple effect stopped there. My husband did not experience any symptoms of PTS from helping me through the resolution. Think of the significance of one incident of trauma. How far can the ripples go? Why are crisis managers like the fire fighter and like me so intensely affected, and why is it apparently delayed? What are the implications for society at large?! Let us look at the way the existential identity of a crisis manager is affected by trauma, both directly and indirectly.

Crisis Manager examples include:

- Police, Probation, Parole and Correctional Officers
- Social workers
- Judges, Lawyers and Other Officers of the Court
- Emergency Medical Personnel and Fire Fighters

- Military Personnel
- Pastoral, Grief, Rape, Chemical and Co-dependency Counselors
- Psychotherapists
- Teachers, Nurses
- Educational, Medical and Law Enforcement Administrators

Organizations that have been created to deal with crisis management include:

- The Courts
- Legislature
- Community Executive (local, state, federal) Management
- Hospitals
- Schools
- Women's Shelters
- Churches
- Law Enforcement Agencies
- The Military
- Child Protective Services
- Chemical and Codependency Programs

Crisis managers can be affected by trauma directly and indirectly. Examples of direct trauma would be a police officer's being shot or shot at, shooting a suspect, finding a murder victim, etc. Examples of indirect trauma would be a counselor or pastor listening to stories of horrific abuse or death.

Psychological trauma for most people is a rapid and destructive change to their personal identities. For crisis managers, however, it is a little more complicated. As we have discussed in previous chapters, the personal or Existential identity is made up of a person's values, beliefs, images and reality. Non-crisis managers operate out of this personal identity, and psychological trauma affects this personal identity. Crisis managers, however, operate out of two identities simultaneously—their personal identities and their professional identities. Therefore, crisis managers have a unique problem. This problem develops when trauma causes a rapid and destructive change to their identities and the professional identity assimilates the change but the personal identity does not. This problem is made even more complicated when the professional identity denies that the damage to the personal identity has occurred. This is when the professional crisis manager says to himself or herself, "That's life. That's my job. Some make it, some don't. I won't let it get to *me*."

The consequences of leaving any psychological trauma unaddressed are deterioration of both of the identities and inevitable erosion, if not complete breakdown, of both personal and professional management control.

Remember, identity is made up of four things: values, beliefs, images and reality. Since the crisis manager has two identities, personal and professional, he or she has two sets of values, two sets of beliefs, two sets of images and two realities.

When psychological trauma contradicts values and beliefs, damage occurs to the personal identity. The professional identity of the crisis manager remains intact, since it is a function of his or her job requirement. For example, when a soldier—trained to fight and kill—shoots another human being, professionally he or she has done what he or she is supposed to do, and therefore the professional identity not only remains intact but is supported and reinforced. However, a basic personal belief is that human life is something to be preserved and protected. That may be one of the main reasons the soldier joined the military. Therefore, the personal identity is being contradicted and is torn apart. This is experienced internally, even unconsciously, and results in loss and emotional pain.

Left unaddressed, this damage will result in personal behavioral change. Initially, the behavioral change may be slight and not noticeable at all professionally. Many police dramas on television demonstrate this quite effectively. The police officer has to shoot someone at work, goes home and is quiet and distant from his family. Eventually, the distance grows; the family feels isolated and may result in the wife's asking for a divorce or the children's acting out to get attention. The crisis manager may even become violent, acting out his repressed pain and loss. The same things happened which were described in earlier chapters: the loss chains formed, the streaming of emotion occurred, the escalation and expansion of emotion took place. The problems snowballed and the personal identity became torn to shreds. During the first few weeks, months or even years of the trauma's expansion into the personal identity, the professional identity remains undisturbed. In fact, in many cases the response to the deteriorating personal identity is the strengthening of the professional identity. The person pours himself or herself into his or her work, even appearing heroic in character. That is why the families of many crisis managers, including pastors and counselors, wonder, "How can they think he is so wonderful at work when he's so horrible to us at home?" The family is very confused and hurt, especially since it does not appear to be affecting his work. No one there sees the difference. Therefore, the family is not supported when reaching out for help to the source of employment.

Eventually, the influence of the trauma on the personal identity begins to affect the professional identity and behavioral changes occur at work, also. These may include:

- confused thought and erratic behavior,
- wide emotional swings,
- inflexible and inaccurate interpretations of rules, guidelines and laws,
- fusion with victims,
- burnout,
- alignment with perpetrators,
- impaired judgment,
- illegal or unethical use of power,
- social self-destruction,
- And even suicide.

These changes in professional behavior contradict professional values, beliefs, images and reality and result in loss and pain in the professional identity.

Stop Treating Symptoms and Start Resolving Trauma!

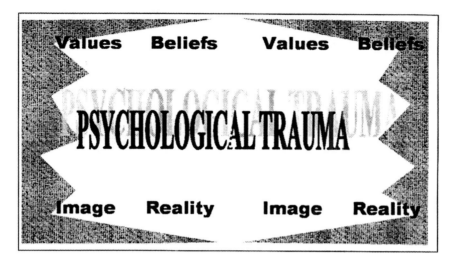

Figure 35 - The contradictions to professional values, beliefs, image and reality result in the trauma's expansion into Professional Identity

If this goes unaddressed, the trauma can destroy both the personal and professional identity and will, inevitably, influence the organization. The most recent term used for this is "compassion fatigue," formerly known as burnout. It does not have to be this way, however. While psychological trauma is a rapid and destructive change to identity, the resolution of trauma is a reconciliation or successful assimilation of that change. For crisis managers, trauma resolution *must* include recognition of both the personal and professional identities and any effects the trauma may have had on them, respectively.

Naturally, if the trauma to the crisis manager's personal identity were to be resolved *before* it spreads into the professional identity, the destruction to the professional identity could be prevented altogether. If the trauma's influence has already spread into the professional identity, it too can be resolved and the psychological/physiological damage reversed. However, certain tangible losses, such as family, career, ranking, etc, may never be regained exactly as before. Thus it is better to resolve the trauma before it spreads and causes further damage.

Using a proactive approach will prevent the development of further trauma. By *proactive* I mean an approach that does not wait on symptoms to appear; an approach that assumes the damage to the personal identity has been done because the trauma has occurred; I mean Trauma Resolution Therapy.

A modified form of TRT is used for Crisis Managers when the trauma experienced on the job is recent (within the last 90 days). There are six basic steps.

1. Identify the trauma-causing event.

2. Describe the trauma-causing event;

   a. orally,

   b. in writing (if necessary or helpful),

   c. follow the TRT Phase One format.

3. Identify and express feelings or emotional states:

   a. orally,

   b. in writing (if necessary or helpful),

   c. follow the TRT Phase One format (i.e., process the feelings existentially).

4. Identify values and beliefs contradicted by the traumatic episode:

   a. orally,

   b. in writing (if necessary and/or helpful).

5. Identify losses directly resulting from contradicted values identified in Step 4:

   a. orally,

   b. in writing (if necessary and/or helpful).

6. Reflect, affirm and facilitate the manager's identifying, acknowledging and accepting his or her true value.

Notice that most of the work can be done either orally or in writing. The oral work is done in the first meeting when the trauma is recent. If it is particularly horrific, a follow-up session or sessions may be done with the crisis manager's writing out the information between the sessions. If the oral method is used for a recent event, resolution may take place in 30 minutes. More horrific events or events that occurred more than 90 days prior to the session, giving them time to expand their influence on the personal and/or professional identity, will take longer.

The authors of *An Etiotropic Trauma Management System for Crisis Managers,* Jesse Collins, Nancy Carson, and Craig Carson, list five guidelines for the implementation of such a program. They are:

1. Resolve the trauma. Do not focus on symptoms. Focus on facilitating personnel exposed to trauma into TRT as soon as time allows. Centering the program around the manifestations of the trauma's symptoms means centering the program around destruction.

2. The referral process must be active as opposed to passive. Self-referral management approaches will play into the trauma's defense structure (professional stoicism). In trauma cases, if the program waits for the victim to discover his or her need for assistance, timely resolution will be prevented. Destruction is highly probable.

3. Never attempt to resolve crisis-manager trauma for the purpose of correcting professional behavior. If the goal is anything other than to resolve the trauma, TRT will not be effective.

4. Address the trauma directly. Do not become diverted by other issues (except of course, where incidents of chemical dependency or mental illness are discovered and have to be addressed).

5. Refer even the toughest crisis manager for trauma resolution despite his or her strength of character. Strength of character is not an adequate defense against internal destruction from psychological trauma. Usually, the stronger the character, the greater the internal damage.[21]

Military Personnel

In June, 1990, following a U.S. Army Chaplain's study of ETM's clinical and industry system management programs, Jesse Collins, through the ETM Trainer Craig Carson, was requested by leaders of the Army's Chaplain Corps to write a plan with which to test and employ ETM in combat, specifically under guerrilla warfare conditions. Unfortunately, the Gulf War started at the time of the writing, August, 1990, and final acceptance and implementation of the plan were stopped. Most of the participating officers received transfer orders related to the War. When the war was over, many permanent personnel reductions throughout the military brought the plan's prospective implementation to a close. Guerrilla and terrorism combat principles have remained pretty much the same since that earlier time, and our government continues to be substantially weakened by that reality. Jesse has written an ETM thesis and implementation plan for those who would like to overcome guerrilla and terrorist warfare. At the time of this writing, the theory and plan are provided in total in the tutorial section of http://etiotropic.org.

Trauma for crisis managers cannot be avoided; it is their job to deal with trauma. It does not, however, have to take the extreme toll on them that it does. The initial effects to the personal identity can be reversed and the damage to the professional identity prevented with a little time, effort and planning. Even if the work to prevent the damage to the professional identity was not done, there is still hope. The psychological damage to both identities can still be reversed, even years after the incidents have occurred.

Chapter Twelve: Victory! True Stories Of People Overcoming Tragedy In Their Lives

This chapter highlights some of the courageous people I have known who have experienced devastating trauma and overcome it. They have gone on not only to survive but also to flourish. I truly feel blessed to have been a part of their lives for a short time. The names have been changed along with any other significant identifying information. I am sorry if anyone reads this and thinks it is about him or her, but since so much identifying information has been changed, most likely it is not.

Anna

Some of Anna's story is told in the first chapter. Her marriage to Jim was not only a disappointment but also almost deadly. She experienced five years of severe abuse that was physical, sexual, verbal, and emotional. She finally left him because she knew that he was planning to murder her and then kill himself. Before leaving him, however, she went to a pastor for counsel. She was told by this well-meaning pastor that divorcing her husband was wrong and that God would never approve. Unfortunately, she did not tell the pastor the gruesome details of her abuse, and he did not ask. She felt horribly guilty but decided that she would rather live than die. She had developed a potentially life threatening disease but had gone without treatment, hoping that she would just die and not have to go through a divorce.

She left Jim, started a new career and heard about Trauma Resolution Therapy from a seminar I led in a small town. She entered individual therapy and eventually group therapy. She wrote all *forty* of her Phase One incidents in one weekend. She read during her first week in group, something I do not usually allow. For the first few months, Anna showed little emotion during her reading. The group would be left feeling devastated, but Anna would say, "I feel a little irritated." She became fearful that this therapy would not work. I encouraged her to just continue reading, let the feelings come, and not try to force them. Soon she was showing appropriate emotion, weeping during group, and expressing intense anger at Jim. As she moved through the phases, her energy level increased and her depression subsided. She no longer wanted to die and began to see herself with a future.

Anna continues in her new career, happy, content and praying for a new husband. She is content to remain single and now truly believes that God is on her side.

Sarah

I met Sarah at a seminar on sexual abuse, which I was conducting at a church. She came to counseling because she was in a homosexual relationship, believed it was wrong, and thought she wanted out. Sarah had grown up in a fine Christian home, with loving parents and well-adjusted siblings. Unfortunately, she was sexually abused multiple times by an older male cousin whom she adored. After several years of marriage, she became involved with another woman, divorced her husband, and immersed herself in the gay lifestyle. Her current gay lover was also abusive. Sarah entered individual therapy and eventually group therapy. It was very difficult for her to admit to the other women in the group that she was writing about a homosexual relationship, but she did. Through TRT and individual therapy she saw major changes. Unknown to me at the time, she continued in the homosexual relationship for several months during her initial counseling. Because of her faithfulness in heading in the right direction, however, God started rearranging her life. He sent her parents, who were unaware of her lesbian lifestyle, to live with near her. She confessed to them what she had been doing and told them of the childhood sexual abuse. They were shocked but remained loving and supportive. She became accountable to them. She had lost a lot of money and had debt due to the abusive homosexual relationship in which she had been involved. She ended the relationship for good and committed to an abstinent lifestyle. Her Phase Five B project was extremely touching. She came to group in her "lesbian" style clothes—something about which we as a group had totally forgotten. We had not noticed the gradual change in her dress as it became increasingly feminine and stylish. She played a Christian tape and had a suitcase that she laid on the floor. As the song played, she slowly took off the clothes and placed them in the suitcase. Underneath were her new, feminine clothes. After placing everything in the suitcase, she closed it up, handed it to me and said, "Denice, I don't need these anymore. Will you throw them away for me?" With tears running down my face, I said I would be happy to do it. I went out and threw the case in the garbage. Everyone was crying. The change in her was amazing! It had happened so gradually that we had not realized how drastic it was until that night. Sarah went on to complete TRT on the child sexual abuse with as much success.

Dana

I first met Dana when she was admitted into our Christian inpatient program. She was very depressed and experiencing severe flashbacks. She would be reminded of something her stepfather had done and go into a transient psychotic state where she felt and believed that she was experiencing the sexual abuse right then. She had horrible nightmares of his torturous abuse. She started writing her Phase One incidents while in the hospital but continued in outpatient therapy group. She continued to experience flashbacks for a short while, but as she continued to write, read in group, and process her feelings, they went away. She told horrible stories of how her stepfather tortured her with various objects while molesting her. She told of at least one incident where he tied her up out in the woods, and he and several of his friends had sex with her. Her processing included much intense crying, wailing, and shredding of magazines. She got so angry she could break the back of a magazine with one twist of her small hands. As she moved through the phases, I could literally see a peace coming over her. Toward the end of her phases, she and her husband decided that he should accept a job offer in another state. Some amazing events took place as to the timing of their house's selling, finding a house in the new town, and finishing her TRT at the right time. Truly amazing was a totally unexpected series of events. Dana had not had contact with her real father since she was a child. She found where he lived and contacted him. He lived only a short distance from their new town. He welcomed her phone call warmly, met her and helped them find a house. He apologized for his neglect and explained that his ex-wife had threatened him if he came around. They developed a new relationship in которой a lot of healing took place, totally unexpectedly. When we are faithful to do what God asks of us, it is amazing how He goes to work and brings things together of which we could have never dreamed.

Bob and Alice

Bob came in with his wife who was saying she was ready to leave. This was his second marriage and he did not want another ruined marriage. While on a work assignment, he had left with a co-workers car and gone to buy crack. Several days later, some friends from his church tracked him down. He was in a hotel, smoking crack and totally wasted. He lost his job and was about to lose his wife. This would not be the first time he had lost everything to crack. He started in the six-month sobriety program and Alice started in a non-CD TRT women's group. He moved on to a men's CD group a few months later. He blamed his parents and was convinced he had childhood trauma. I was convinced he did not. He had 26+ years of drug usage, including alcohol; various illegal drugs, prescription drugs and his drug of choice—crack. Through much assistance from his church, he participated in some sobriety groups and maintained his sobriety. Alice completed her five phases on his drug abuse and went on to some past trauma—pre-Bob. Eventually, Bob contacted his parents, invited them over and apologized for the money, dignity and things he had stolen from them. Now, he was convinced he did not have childhood trauma. It took him a couple of years to finish his TRT on his chemical abuse, but he did finish it! He and his wife stood before their church and testified to the grace of God. It was a miracle.

Janice

Janice was referred by a school counselor due to her six-year-old daughter's having problems in school. I did short-term, goal-focused therapy with the daughter and she improved quickly. I also worked with Janice on parenting skills. In the assessment, Janice discussed her own experiences growing up with an alcoholic father and her fear of inappropriately parenting her daughter. She had become obsessed with her only child's every move. I recommended TRT, but she was not interested at the time. They left therapy and came back about a year later, but this time Janice came for herself. She had started back to school and became obsessed with getting perfect grades. She wept, she worried, she struggled over her college classes, and she wondered if it was all worth it. Her marriage had become boring and tedious, and she did not know what to do. After several sessions I again suggested TRT. This time she hesitantly agreed to try it for a while. Initially she said there were very few incidents of her father's behavior that she could remember. He was not violent or mean—he was disgusting, pitiful, and weepy when he was drunk. He was also drunk most of the time. After her first readings in individual therapy she was shocked at the emotion that came up inside of her, since she had become convinced that her childhood was no big deal. She entered group therapy, and as she heard others read, she remembered even more incidents with her father. She had at least twenty-five incidents before she finished. When she entered TRT, she was very tense, obsessed with school and her daughter's behavior, very focused on her husband and angry at him much of the time. She had been raised in a Catholic church but had never been particularly spiritual. When she left TRT, she was like a different person. She laughed a lot more, she stopped worrying about school and finished with great—although not perfect—grades. She reported that she felt as if she "had been walking around in a fog all of her life and suddenly the fog had lifted." Her relationships with people became much less obsessive and more fun. She reported that she felt "free." I have heard from her once or twice since then. She called to say thank you and that she was doing great. Life was not perfect, as her mother developed breast cancer and her sister divorced, but she was handling it well. Her spiritual life improved also. She began praying again, determined the difference between right and wrong rather than letting society dictate it for her, and even started going to church.

Nora

Nora was referred by a friend. She initially came to see me before I started using TRT. She came for various reasons and left when she felt she had accomplished enough. Eventually, she remarried and came back with her husband, for they were having marital problems. This time I convinced her to deal with the past trauma. Both her mother and her father were alcoholics. She first wrote about her mother in Phase One, then she wrote about her father in Phase One. She combined them for Phases Two through

Five. She described a very wretched childhood. Her mother would be gone days at a time while on a drunken binge. She would find her mother in all sorts of disgusting and filthy situations and take responsibility to clean her up and take care of her. Her parents were both arrested for fighting and public drunkenness. She became the true caretaker of herself and her little brother. Even after she became an adult, her mother continued to drink and embarrass her at work, at home, and in public. At one point in Phase One she had to list all of the names that her mother called her and use the sentence stem "You called me a …." She had two full pages! When she started the group Nora had a tough, street wise, shell. As she progressed she visibly softened. Her face softened and she even looked younger. After completing her five phases, she was much happier in her marriage, though I cannot say that the marital problems resolved themselves. She made some changes on her own, but her husband did not. As far as I know, they are still married, but how happily I do not know.

Bethany

Bethany also started seeing me prior to my involvement with TRT. She participated in one of my women's survivor groups when they were unstructured. She focused on her father's sexual abuse until her husband ended up in the hospital for alcoholism. She left therapy for several years and returned due to her husband's continued use of alcohol and her serious thoughts of divorce. This time I convinced her to write about her husband. Although she initially thought she had very little to write about, she came up with twenty or more episodes. As she progressed, she would tell me how she was increasingly setting more appropriate boundaries with her husband and with other people in her life. After graduating from the group, she called back to report that her husband had quit drinking, even though he did not want to, that their marriage had improved, and that she felt much better about her life in general.

Terry and David

Terry and David came to see me for marital counseling. He had a history of drug use and had been sexually abused. He had recently received an injury on the job and was involved in a court case. Terry started in her TRT, slowly writing about David. David did not do much. He kept disappearing for days at a time, then would return, repent and admit to drug use. Eventually, Terry figured out he was involved in pornography and having a relationship with a woman he met on the internet. The police became involved due to his increasing violence. A member from Terry's group ended up involved when she passed Terry chasing David in a vehicle he had stolen from her home after he left. What a mess! Terry hung in there and kept writing. She became increasingly strong and was able to send David packing for good. She finished her TRT and went on to minister to other hurting women, using TRT.

Mark

Mark was referred by a psychiatrist following several months of medication treatment which had not resolved his problems. You read about him in Chapter Two—he experienced an industrial accident. Mark had no other sources of trauma and entered a co-ed TRT survivors' group to read about the industrial accident. He had withdrawn from his previously close family and felt depressed and anxious all of the time. He could not bring himself to return to work at the plant, yet he could not make a move in another direction. He had minimal individual or couples' therapy. Upon completing his five-phase process, Mark noted a marked improvement in his relationship with his wife and his son. Although he did not return to his previous employment, he made specific plans to start a new business on his own. Mark was part of my only co-ed group and contributed a lot to the group process. Since his graduation, however, I have stuck with women's or men's groups.

Barbara

Barbara began seeing me following her attendance at a lay counseling class I taught at her church. She was obviously very angry. She had been hurt by a previous unlicensed counselor and had a lot of difficulty trusting me. We did a lot of individual therapy prior to my beginning to use TRT. As we started into the TRT process, it was obvious she had many sources of trauma. I learned a lot from Barbara. Her marriage was a great source of pain for her. She denied any physical abuse except one incident, during which they were arguing when he pushed her and she fell down the stairs. She was very focused on the fact that her daughter had been sexually abused many years earlier, and Barbara had recently told her husband about their daughter's abuse.

We wrote about her daughter's abuse first. Then we went on to write about her own sexual abuse from a male cousin as she grew up. During this time she was listening to others read in the group about their husbands' abusing them. She began to recall other incidents in which her husband had abused her. As she began writing about him, she ended up with thirty or more very violent episodes of abuse. Although she had previously shown a decrease in survival responses, she became increasingly angry as she wrote. She had also changed to another individual therapist, due to my being absent for a while on maternity leave. She got intensely angry, and she directed a lot of it at me and the group. One day she decided to quit group.

If I had it to do over again, I would have had her write about her husband first, even if she did not want to do it. As she began to write what she did remember, more would have surfaced. As it was, she was on her third source of trauma and she was exhausted. Even though she quit at the end of Phase One, I included her in this victory chapter because she is victorious. Although she has not resolved all of the trauma in her past, she did resolve some of it. Someday, I hope she finishes the rest.

Karen

Some friends at her church who were personally familiar with the TRT process referred Karen. When she came to see me, she was obviously out of control with her anger. She and her young son fought all of the time, and she could not seem to control her rages. She would call me in a crisis, fighting with her son, and then get angry at me. She had grown up with an alcoholic father who became an outlaw biker. As she wrote her Phase One incidents, it became very clear to me why she was so angry. Frankly, I was surprised that she was doing as well as she was. As a teenager, she witnessed a drunken orgy put on by her father's biker gang, which included the gang rape of another teenage girl. Once when she was visiting him from out of state, her father abandoned her in the middle of a large city with only his van to sleep in, no food, and no money. Physical abuse, vulgarity, and slave labor were common place. Her list of losses in Phase Two and Four were *pages* long. She spent a lot of time crying and shredding magazines (our answer to hitting pillows or hitting chairs with bats). Her relationship with her daughter improved tremendously. Her parenting skills became much more appropriate. After she finished Phase Four I became concerned, however, because I had not seen the usual reduction in anger. After she finished Phase Five A, I found out why.

Several more incidents had come to mind that she had not written about at all. She was extremely frustrated but nevertheless followed my direction and wrote them in Phase One style, then carried them forward through all of the other Phases until she was back to Phase Five B. Then the reduction in anger became obvious. Even her features noticeably softened, and she looked younger. Unfortunately, it also became clear to her that she would have to write about a former boyfriend who was an addict and very abusive. Eventually, she returned to complete her second, and last, source of trauma.

This is just a *very small* sampling of the people I have personally had the opportunity to introduce to TRT. If you were reading this book and did not see your story in here, please do not be offended! Writing everyone's story would take a couple of more books! Write your story down and send it to me. I will put it in the next book. Thanks for reading!

Denice Colson

Appendix A: Trauma Assessment

Many people realize that past trauma of some type is affecting their current lives. On the other hand, many people have no idea why they struggle with current problems and see no connection with their past trauma. Not all problems in peoples' lives are caused by past trauma. We are imperfect people living in an imperfect world. We make bad choices, and we sin. We rebel, and sometimes we just do not care what the consequences are. Many experiences in life are traumatic but would not necessarily be defined as "trauma" for the purpose of TRT. If there is trauma in your past, however, resolving it is important. The following questions and statements will help to explore whether you have trauma that needs resolving.

As a child:

- Did you ever experience inappropriate touching of a sexual nature, or touching that made you feel self-conscious or uncomfortable?

- Were you ever punished by a parent with hitting that left bruises or bleeding?

- Did you ever think that your parents were abusive? Why?

- Did your parents ever call you insulting names like "stupid," "brat," "bitch," "creep," or any others you can recall?

- Did anyone in your house get drunk? Use drugs? (Including pain medications, Valium and other sedating prescription medications.)

- Did anyone in your house get violent, hitting things, throwing things, hitting people, breaking things, etc.?

- Were you or anyone in your home involved in a serious accident?

- Was anyone in your home diagnosed with a mental illness?

- Was anyone in your home physically or sexually abused? Did you witness it?

- Were you threatened by or did you experience a natural catastrophe, such as major earthquakes, hurricanes, floods, typhoons, tornados, etc.

- Did either of your parents serve in the military? Was he or she ever in battle? Was he or she diagnosed with Post-Traumatic Stress Disorder or anything similar?

- Did you use drugs or alcohol?

- Did you or anyone in your family attempt suicide? Did anyone succeed? Did you witness it?

<u>As an adult (answer the previous questions as well as the following):</u>

- Do you live with or are you involved with someone who might have a drinking or drug problem?

- Have you been in a relationship where someone hit you when he or she was angry, drunk, or out of sorts?

- Do you use alcohol on a regular basis?

- Have you been in a relationship with someone who insulted you by calling you names, making faces or gestures?

- Have you had an abortion or, if you are a man, has your wife or girlfriend had an abortion?

- Has your spouse or former spouse had an affair?

- Has your spouse divorced you against your will?

- Have you experienced the sudden/premature/unexpected death of a loved one?

- Have you given birth to a child with a birth defect?

- Have you or a loved one had a terminal or life-threatening illness?

- Have you used alcohol or drugs to the extent that someone close to you worried about your use? Have you received a DUI?

- Have you viewed pornography on a regular basis? Have you visited strip clubs or solicited prostitutes? Have you or someone else you love been concerned or even angry about your involvement with any of these types of things?

- Have you been diagnosed as anorexic or bulimic?

- Have you ever gambled compulsively?

- Have you or do you work as a crisis manager and experience primary or secondary traumatic incidents?

If you answered yes to any of the above, you have experienced trauma and may have etiology (contradicted identity-values, beliefs, image and reality). You are most likely experiencing some survival responses related to loss and pain repressed in your subconscious. The extent of the damage must be assessed by a trained counselor certified in the use of Trauma Resolution Therapy. No matter how severe, all traumas deserve the opportunity to be resolved. If you have experienced trauma and have not been through a structured resolution process, it does affect

Appendix B: Etiotropic Trauma Management FAQ'S

Q: What does Etiotropic mean?

A: It means that the assessment and treatment activities all focus on the "etiology" of the trauma. "Etiology" means the source or cause of a disease or problem. In this case, ETM theory states that the etiology of the trauma is contradicted existential identity. Your "existential identity" is made up of your values, beliefs, image and reality. So for example, if my husband gets drunk and acts like an idiot in public, many of my values, beliefs, images and reality will be contradicted. I believe that getting drunk is dangerous and wrong. My image of my husband is of a steady, sober man who also believes that getting drunk is wrong. I value trustworthiness, stability and the opinions of others. Therefore, my husband's toxic (drunk) behavior contradicts my existential identity. If it goes unresolved, this will be the continuous source or etiology of my trauma.

Q: What is Trauma Resolution Therapy (TRT)?

A: Trauma Resolution Therapy (TRT) is the application of ETM theory. It is a five phase structured process for resolving trauma at the source. All aspects of TRT support keeping the focus of the work on the etiology until the etiology is reversed i.e., the trauma is resolved. The five written phases can be completed in individual or group settings. There is a long form and a short form of TRT. The long form (five structured phases) is applied to long term trauma. Long-term trauma refers to trauma or a series of related traumas that occurred at least more than 90 days ago, but usually many years ago. The short form is applied to near term trauma which has occurred within the last 90 days. It involves using only phases 1, 2 and 5. There is also a crisis management tool used with crisis managers who have experienced on the job trauma either directly or indirectly.

Q: How long has ETM been around?

A: It was created in the early 1980's by husband and wife team Jesse Collins and Nancy Carson while they were developing and managing several substance abuse treatment facilities in Texas. It grew out of their need to find a more effective way of treating the addicted patients and their family members. Through much study and research the Five Phase Model of TRT evolved. In the mid-1980's, the oil bust caused them to lose funding for their facilities and they transitioned into training. Craig Carson, a therapist working with them at the time, took on the task of training while Jesse and Nancy developed the curriculum. Over a thousand counselors, social workers, and other personnel have been trained in this method in Texas, Louisiana and Georgia.

Q: How does the TRT approach to treating trauma, or PTSD, differ from other approaches?

A: All aspects of TRT keep the focus on the etiology or source of the trauma rather than the symptoms. The opposite of Etiotropic is Nosotropic. Nosotropic means that the focus is on the reduction of symptoms. While all treatment occurs on a continuum, TRT is the only fully Etiotropic method for resolving trauma. Behavioral methods include behavior modification, medication, and systematic desensitization. All of these are fully nosotropic in that their only goal is to reduce the symptoms of PTSD or chronic stress responses. Cognitive-behavioral methods spend some time on developing insight into the source of the symptoms but only to figure out a way to reduce the symptoms. Psychodynamic models start out by delving into the etiology, but again to identify symptoms that need to be changed. TRT, on the other hand, maintains the focus on the etiology, even precluding attempts to change symptoms, until the etiology is fully reversed. ETM theory sees symptoms as a normal and necessary response to trauma and believes that the focus on reducing symptoms not only does not work in the long-run, but can increase etiology or damage to the existential identity. It can actually make things worse.

Q: Can this be used in couple's therapy?

A: ETM/TRT can be used conjointly with couple's therapy and in unique cases, directly in couple's therapy. Let me explain. The sole purpose of TRT is to resolve trauma. Not to increase communication effectiveness, teach appropriate boundaries, etc. These are the goals of traditional couple's therapy. Following the guidelines, couples can participate in their separate TRT processes and come together on a more sporadic schedule for basic couples counseling. The guidelines are that the individual TRT must always take precedence and limited progress can be expected in couples counseling until the individual TRT processes have moved past phase 2. On certain occasions, assessment shows that a couple is experiencing current or recent trauma from the same source, usually a teenage or adult child with some type of addiction. In these cases, the couple can move through the five phase TRT process, both focusing on the child (or source of trauma) and do so together in a joint session. In other words, they form their own little two person TRT group.

Q: Not to be selfish, but as a Counselor, how can adopting the TRT/ETM methods help me?

A: Not a selfish question at all. We should use methods that work for us as well as our clients. It has many benefits. I discovered all of these when I started using TRT in my private outpatient practice and inpatient practice in 1991.

1. It makes sense. It is logical and easy to explain to clients. Clients like it. When I sold my Bellaire, Texas practice in 1998 to move with my family to Georgia, I had 3 outpatient TRT groups running (as well as all of my individual, family and couples work). Two of these groups were women's groups and one was a CD men's group. I sold my practice to a male therapist who was also trained in TRT. Since most of my clients were female who had specifically sought out a female therapist you would normally think "Bad move!" However, we did not lose one client due to the transition from female to male! Why? Because they all believed in the TRT process. They were committed, not to me, but to completing the five phase process. They had seen it work both in their own lives and in the lives of their fellow group members. Many of my referrals came from satisfied customers. So much so that I had to keep starting new groups or finding some way to keep certain people apart. Finally, I just started telling people you'll have to be

in a group with someone you know from church, Bible study, etc. I would only keep family members (sisters, spouses) separate.

2. It's economical. While the TRT process starts out in individual sessions, normally it progresses to group. Group size is usually limited to 6-8 individuals. However, you can charge a much lower fee and still collect more for a 1 ½ hour group session than you would for an individual session. I had some very low paying clients and occasionally even a pro-bono client. Putting them into group just made sense.

3. The client doesn't become focused on you for all the answers. Now some therapists like this sense of power. If so, this would be a negative for you, not a positive. The function of the counselor in the TRT process is one of "facilitator". Your role is to keep the client focused on following the structure. Other than that, you offer encouragement and treatment planning. In a group setting, clients begin to depend on the structure and on each other. Clients will call each other to find out how to write a phase 2 incident before calling me, many times. Clients will offer to help each other write a phase they have already completed. I do not become the center of their lives. I like that! By using TRT you are truly working your way out of a job, as it should be in this field.

4. By becoming certified in ETM, you could market yourself in your community as an expert in trauma recovery. This can open up entirely new referral sources for you. There are planned lectures you can use or adapt for community presentations. Education is a very important part of the TRT process. While a minimal amount is needed to prepare clients to participate in the group or individual process, the more education you offer, the faster your client becomes committed to the process and the more family members you will have participating.

5. There is a beginning and an ending. In grad school, this was a question we all wrestled with. When do you know when you are done? Usually we leave that up to the client. If they don't show up and don't return your phone calls, they're done. Some clients have the means to stay in counseling for the better part of their adult lives. TRT starts with assessment, moves from phase 1-5 in a logical progression, and when phase 5b is complete, they are done. They can leave, and they know it. If they have another

source of trauma to work on, you'll know it and so will they. After a break, they can start again following the same logical process. Clients like this idea. I like this idea!

Q: How long does the TRT process take to complete?

A: When people hear that this is a five phase process, they sometimes think "Oh, I can get this done in 5 weeks??" No, TRT is not necessarily quick. The short-form for near-term trauma and the crisis management model are quick, usually less than ten sessions for the short-form. The crisis management is usually 1-3, 30-45 minute sessions. For long-term trauma, however, it can take anywhere from 6 months to 2 years. The longest I have had was 2 ½ years. It depends on the severity of the trauma, how many incidents the client recalls, how diligently they write, how consistently they attend their prescribed sessions, and the unknown factor. Will they have to move out of town? Will they have another baby? Will they get sick? Part of the applied structure is that we work on one source of trauma at a time, beginning with the most recent or most pressing. After completing this, we move in a chronologically descending order, allotting a full 5 phases to each source until they are all completed. Full recovery from all trauma is finished when all sources or trauma have been completed.

Q: Is TRT a Christian Counseling technique?

A: ETM and TRT are not specifically Christian, just like antibiotics are not specifically Christian. However, there is nothing in the theory or methodology that contradicts scripture. In fact, TRT supports many directives of scripture. TRT goes to the *root* of the problem rather than dealing only with the *fruit*, or symptoms. TRT focuses on changes from the inside, out. In Matthew 23:25, Jesus said:

> *"Woe to you, teachers of the law and Pharisees, you hypocrites! You clean the outside of the cup and dish, but inside they are full of greed and self-indulgence. Blind Pharisee! First clean the inside of the cup and dish, and then the outside also will be clean."*

Of course, Jesus was talking about sin in the heart. That we can look great on the outside, but inside have hearts full of hate. However, this principle of changing from the inside out summarizes the approach of Trauma Resolution Therapy. First resolve the trauma at the root or source. The survival responses resulting from the repressed loss and pain will drop away on their own when they are no longer needed. TRT puts structure to the mandate to "bear one another's burdens", and to "weep with those who weep". It puts a structure to coming along beside someone and going through the grief and loss with them.

Q: How can I become certified in Etiotropic Trauma Management?

A: You must participate in a certification workshop in person or on-line. You can contact Denice Colson of Trauma Education & Consultation Services at 404-317-3844 or by email at Denice@TraumaEducation.com. You can visit the TECS website at www.TraumaEducation.com.

Q: Who qualifies to be certified in Etiotropic Trauma Management?

A: ANYONE willing to participate in the training process can receive some level of certification in ETM. Since ETM is actually an *accounting* program for trauma and not a psychotherapy--(Dictionary.com definition: The treatment of mental and emotional disorders through the use of psychological techniques designed to encourage communication of conflicts and insight into problems, with the goal being relief of symptoms, changes in behavior leading to improved social and vocational functioning, and personality growth.)—even lay-people can be certified. There are, however, two levels of certification. Level 1: Certification (full) is for people who are otherwise licensed by their state to perform counseling and psychotherapy services. Level 2: Associate Certification is for lay-persons who are not otherwise licensed to offer counseling and psychotherapy services. They are limited to use under their state laws and requested to seek regular supervision from a fully certified TRT professional. They are limited to certification in TRT techniques only. This does not certify them to perform marital counseling or any other specialized form of counseling or psychotherapy.

Endnotes

[1] For a note about abortion please see Chapter Four: *Survival Responses*, category number three, Aggressive type.

[2] Collins, Jesse and Nancy Carson. <u>TRT Educational Program Presenter's Handbook</u>. 1992.

[3] Collins, Jesse and Nancy Carson. <u>TRT Educational Program Presenter's Handbook</u>. 1992.

[4] Collins, Jesse and Nancy Carson. <u>TRT Educational Program Presenter's Handbook</u>. 1992.

[5] Collins, Jesse and Nancy Carson. <u>TRT Educational Program Presenter's Handbook</u>. 1992.

[6] <u>Webster's New Collegiate Dictionary</u>. 1977.

[7] Collins, Jesse and Nancy Carson. <u>TRT Educational Program Presenter's Handbook</u>. 1992.

[8] Collins, Jesse and Nancy Carson. <u>TRT Educational Program Presenter's Handbook</u>. 1992.

[9] Bremner, J. Douglas. <u>Does Stress Damage the Brain?</u> New York, NY, 2002.

[10] Collins, Jesse. Neurobiology of Psychological Trauma Etiology and Its Reversal with Etiotropic Trauma Management. 2003

[11] Berne, Eric. Games People Play. New York, NY, 1992.

[12] See the definition in Chapter Two, *Understanding The Influence Trauma Has Had On Your Life*

[13] Collins, Jesse and Carson, Nancy. TRT Educational Program Presenters Handbook. 1992.

[14] Ibid.

[15] Collins, Jesse and Carson, Nancy. TRT Educational Program Presenters Handbook. 1992

[16] *The Contemporary English [computer file], electronic ed., Logos Library System*, (Nashville: Thomas Nelson) 1997, c1995 by the American Bible Society.

[17] *The King James Version*, (Cambridge: Cambridge) 1769.

[18] Collins, Jesse and Nancy Carson. TRT Educational Program Presenter's Handbook. 1992.

[19] Kubler-Ross, Elisabeth. On Death and Dying New York:, NY. 1969.

[20] Smalley, Gary. Making Love Last Forever. New York, NY.1996.

[21] Carson, Craig, Jesse Collins and Nancy Carson. TRT Educational Program Presenter's Handbook. 1992.

About the Author

In 1992 Denice Adcock Colson was sitting in her office with a client who said, "You've helped me a lot, but I feel stuck". Denice agreed and added, "Honestly, I don't know what to do about it." A week later Denice was introduced to Etiotropic Trauma Management. Since launching her career in 1982, she had searched for a truly effective way of helping clients put their trauma behind them, but could not get beyond merely helping them manage their symptoms. By the second day of training in this innovative technique, she was convinced that her search was over. Denice continues in part-time practice as a Licensed Professional Counselor while also writing, speaking and enjoying her husband and three children.